THE ULTIMATE GUIDE TO MENOPAUSE GUT HEALTH

7 EASY STEPS TO RESTORE YOUR GUT TO IMPROVE DIGESTION, BALANCE HORMONES, STRENGTHEN IMMUNITY AND OPTIMIZE WELL-BEING

HERA BENNETT

CONTENTS

INTRODUCTION

Many women journey on planet Earth, all in search of something. Some want diamonds and bling, others seek love and dream vacations... But most of us only seek the answer to better gut health.

Gail had always loved tending to her garden, enjoying the fresh air and flower fragrances. But once menopause kicked in, uncontrollable bouts of gas and bloating plagued her afternoons. She constantly ran inside, worried her noisy tummy rumbles might scare away even the birds!

Local artist and painter Patty had always been full of life and energy, but as the hormones of menopause kicked in, her digestive system kicked her while she was down. One week her jeans fit perfectly, and the next she could barely button them due to bloating. She felt like crying about her constantly fluctuating pant size —which brought on even more challenges when she had to decide on an outfit.

Marge loved experiencing new cuisines and could always try even the spiciest dishes without issue, but these days it felt like menopause had changed her digestive system's rules. Last week's delectable curry is this week's bout of misery.

Yoga instructor Sasha had her life and practice all figured out... until menopause threw her a curveball. She went from inspiring calm in her students to being a bubbling cauldron of gas pains and anxiety. Finding inner peace became much harder when her digestive system was so erratic.

What do all of these women have in common? You guessed it—menopause and unfavorable gut health symptoms have abruptly interfered with their lives. All of them are facing the unavoidable challenge of implementing change to improve their health and overall well-being. Join us as we progress through this book to discover the stories of many more women with similar experiences.

UNDERSTANDING MENOPAUSE AND GUT HEALTH

Menopause can change how your body digests food and affects your gut health. If this sounds familiar, know that you don't have to suffer from digestion problems just because you're going through menopause.

Many women journey through menopause searching for relief from distressing symptoms like hot flashes, mood changes, and especially the miserable digestive issues that can come with hormonal ups and downs—uncontrollable gas, bloating, constipation or diarrhea, and even newly developed conditions like IBS or acid reflux. What's supposed to be a normal life transition has turned into a gastrointestinal nightmare!

If you're constantly running to the bathroom, avoiding favorite foods, or skipping events due to embarrassment over flatulence and bloating, this book is for you. There will be no more settling for a life of digestive misery. *The Ultimate Guide to Menopause Gut Health* provides a comprehensive, holistic solution.

Through the 7 **RESTORE Steps to Gut Health** in this book, you'll finally find freedom from

- too much gas, bloating, and other unusual bathroom problems.
- the ups and downs of menopause symptoms, such as hot flashes and mood swings.
- weight struggles and lack of energy.
- a weakened immune system and increased health risks.

Here is just a sneak peak of what you will discover:

- Life-changing recipes that will help you transform your digestion and gut health in a matter of days—no more indigestion or stomachaches!
- The secret to understanding and assessing your gut health so you can cultivate a treatment plan that works for you.
- Everything you need to know about how menopause impacts digestive health and how to harness this information to find true relief.
- How to strengthen your gut microbiome and reap the benefits of these soothing changes through simple and effective lifestyle changes.
- Expert advice on how to optimize your immunity and longevity during menopause by supporting a healthy GI tract and beyond.

- A holistic approach to managing your gut health and menopause symptoms that combines both Western and traditional treatment options.
- Weight management strategies that work during menopause, plus how to use a healthy gut microbiome to your advantage when trying to lose weight!
- Bonus tips for embracing your lifelong wellness and health journey during menopause—health and fitness should never be put on the back burner!

And much more!

Instead of just coping, you'll optimize your well-being by nurturing your gut microbiome, balancing your hormones, and boosting your overall vitality during this important life stage. This comprehensive guide will help you mitigate stomach issues and alleviate those pesky menopause symptoms!

Don't let menopause complications weigh you down any longer. This book provides a natural, sustainable path to feeling like yourself again—regular bathroom habits, a calmer hormone balance, renewed energy, and confidence.

Feeling healthy and cultivating confidence shouldn't be compromised during this transformative phase of your life. Maintaining a healthy lifestyle is one of the best ways to age gracefully and continue feeling your best throughout the process. This detailed guide is the key to helping you feel better than ever and start your revitalizing journey toward better gut health and whole-body wellness!

UNDERSTANDING DIGESTIVE HEALTH

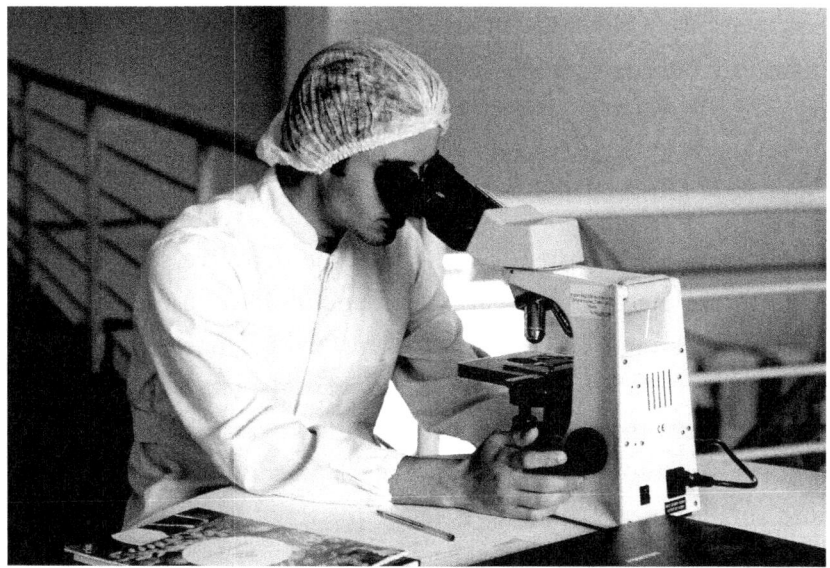

Many women notice changes in their digestion during menopause. This is understandable because of the interconnection of bodily systems and the influence hormonal changes can have on various aspects, including mood and metabolism. Exploring the significance of gut health and digestive wellness during this transitional period is crucial.

Gut Microbiome and Digestion

Gut health generally refers to the balance of microorganisms that thrive in your digestive tract. According to Lynch and Pedersen, these microorganisms—jointly known as the gut microbiome—have a necessary function in digestion and general health (2016). A healthy gut ecosystem can boost nutrient absorption, strengthen immune function, and even influence mood regulation.

Digestive health encompasses a broader scope, including the function of your digestive organs such as the stomach, intestines, liver, pancreas, and gallbladder. Good digestive health implies efficient digestion and absorption of food, timely elimination of waste, and minimal discomfort or dysfunction. Maintaining optimal gut and digestive health is crucial, especially during menopause when changes in hormone levels may disrupt these processes.

Let's take a step-by-step look at how the digestive system functions. Your digestive system starts functioning the moment you anticipate eating (*How the Bowel Works*, n.d.). The smell, sight, or thought of food can make our salivary glands produce saliva, which has enzymes that start breaking down carbohydrates in our mouths. As you chew, your teeth mechanically break down food into smaller pieces, making it easier for the digestive enzymes to do their job.

From your mouth, the chewed food moves down your esophagus through a process called peristalsis—wave-like muscle contractions that push food toward your stomach. Once there, stomach acids and enzymes further break down food into a semi-digested liquid form called chyme. The stomach environment is highly acidic, which helps kill harmful bacteria and activates various digestive enzymes needed to degrade proteins.

Chyme then enters the small intestine, the main site for nutrient absorption. Here, bile from the liver and digestive enzymes from the pancreas mix with the chyme to break down fats, proteins, and carbohydrates. The cells lining your small intestine absorb these nutrients that enter your bloodstream and are transported throughout your body.

The remaining undigested food particles move on to the large intestine where water and electrolytes are absorbed, turning the waste into more solid stool. Your gut microbiome plays an essential role here by fermenting undigested carbohydrates, producing short-chain fatty acids beneficial for colon health. Then the waste is removed through the rectum and anus (*How the Bowel Works*, n.d.).

A complex interplay of hormones and nerves carefully regulates this seamless digestion process. Hormones like gastrin, secretin, and cholecystokinin (CCK) are secreted in response to food intake and regulate various functions such as the release of digestive juices and the movement of food through the GI tract. For instance, CCK signals the gallbladder to release bile into the small intestine while also slowing down gastric emptying so fats can be adequately digested.

Meanwhile, the nervous system ensures that all parts of the digestive system communicate effectively. The enteric nervous system, known as the "second brain," is a large network of nerves located in the walls of the digestive system. It regulates local blood flow, controls muscle contractions for mixing food and moving it forward, and even communicates with the central nervous system for broader regulatory controls.

Understanding these basics allows us to consider the specific issues women face during menopause. Fluctuating estrogen levels can slow peristalsis, leading to symptoms like bloating and constipation (Larson, 2024). Lower estrogen can also disturb the balance of gut microbiota, increasing susceptibility to gut inflammation (Kresser, 2017). Stress, which can be more pronounced during menopause, influences gut health negatively by affecting digestion and altering microbial composition (Kanakiya, 2024).

HOW DIGESTIVE HEALTH AFFECTS OVERALL WELL-BEING

When it comes to the impact of digestive health on overall well-being, it all begins with the strong link between your gut and the rest of your body.

Absorption of Nutrients

To begin with, efficient absorption of nutrients, which directly affects your quality of life, hinges on healthy digestion. When your digestive system is working optimally, you are more likely to experience an increase in energy levels, improved mood, and overall enhanced vitality. It's not just about avoiding discomforts like bloating or indigestion; it's about feeling well enough to actively engage in your daily activities.

Gut Health and Your Immune System

Your gut health significantly influences your immune system. Your gut houses about 70% of your immune system, making it a crucial player in defending your body against pathogens (*What You Should Know*, 2022). A healthy gut supports a balanced immune response, while poor gut health can lead to chronic inflammation and compromised immunity.

Heart Health and Your Gut

Heart health also has significant ties to digestive well-being. Research suggests that the trillions of bacteria residing in your intestines, known as gut microbiota, can impact risk factors for heart disease such as cholesterol and blood pressure (*Gut Check*, 2021). A balanced gut microbiome promotes heart health by reducing inflammation and helping maintain healthy blood lipid levels.

Mental and Emotional Well-Being

Moving on to mental and emotional health, there is increasing evidence supporting the gut-brain axis, which is the bidirectional communication between your gut and brain (Ruder, 2017). This connection explains why digestive issues often coincide with conditions like anxiety or depression. A well-functioning gut can produce and regulate neurotransmitters like serotonin that heavily influence mood and mental stability. This link is so significant that some researchers consider the gut to be our "second brain."

Kidney Health and Digestion

Kidney health is another area where digestive health plays a crit ical role. Kidneys help filter waste from the body, and they need to function well to maintain these balances. Poor digestion can lead to the accumulation of toxins that strain the kidneys, potentially leading to chronic kidney disease. Ensuring your gut is healthy can alleviate undue stress on these vital organs.

Hormones and a Healthy Gut

Hormonal health during menopause is particularly important. Your digestive system helps metabolize hormones and regulate their levels in the body. An unhealthy gut can upset this balance, making menopausal symptoms like hot flashes, mood swings, and weight gain worse. By focusing on maintaining good gut health, you can manage these symptoms more effectively.

Weight Gain and Loss

Both losing and gaining weight are closely connected to gut health. Your digestive system determines how efficiently you metabolize food and store fat. An imbalanced gut flora can lead to weight gain by fostering conditions like insulin resistance. A healthy gut can boost metabolism and support healthier eating habits by signaling satiety to your brain more accurately, helping you avoid overeating.

Investing in Your Digestive Health

Investing in your digestive health yields benefits across various aspects of your overall well-being. It's not just about what occurs in your stomach but how those processes impact your entire body. As you navigate through menopause, pay close attention to your digestive health—it could be the key to managing a range of associated changes and challenges.

Knowing these connections helps you make better decisions about your health. Whether you're considering dietary adjustments, supplements, or lifestyle changes, keep in mind that your gut health is a cornerstone of overall wellness. Consult with your healthcare provider to develop a holistic approach tailored to your unique needs. They can offer specific recommendations based on your health profile to ensure that any steps you take will be both effective and safe.

Achieving and maintaining good gut health requires a thoughtful combination of diet, lifestyle, and possibly medical interventions. Incorporating fiber-rich foods, staying hydrated, reducing stress, and perhaps even exploring probiotics can all contribute to a healthier digestive system.

Focusing on gut health with a new mindset may feel overwhelming. Consistent changes can lead to huge improvements over time. Take a moment to appreciate the incredible work your digestive system does daily, often without much recognition.

When you commit to giving gut health the care and attention it deserves, you're setting yourself up for a healthier, happier life, especially through the life-changing period of menopause. Being proactive now can help ensure that this stage of life is not only manageable but also fulfilling and vibrant.

HOW TO ASSESS YOUR DIGESTIVE HEALTH

When it comes to assessing your digestive health, particularly during menopause and perimenopause, understanding what's happening in your gut can offer a wealth of benefits. This phase of life brings about hormonal fluctuations that can significantly impact your GI system. By knowing how to evaluate your digestive health, you can proactively address issues before they become major concerns.

Signs of a "Not-So-Healthy" Gut

Let's look at the signs of an unhealthy gut and delve into why they occur. These signs range from stomach discomfort, fatigue, and food cravings to more serious issues like unintentional weight changes, skin irritation, allergies, autoimmune conditions, mood issues, and migraines.

Stomach Discomfort

This is often the most immediate indicator of poor gut health. Stomach discomfort can manifest as bloating, gas, or even pain. Such discomfort typically results from imbalances in your gut bacteria, which can be affected by diet, stress, or medications.

Fatigue

This is another common sign of weak gut health and often goes hand in hand with gut issues because a dysfunctional digestive system can lead to poor nutrient absorption.

Food Cravings

Cravings, especially for sugar, can indicate an overgrowth of bad bacteria or yeast, which thrive on sugar. Unintentional weight changes—whether gaining or losing weight—might suggest that your body isn't properly absorbing nutrients or has too much inflammation. For instance, increased inflammation can make it harder to lose weight, while poor absorption can lead to weight loss.

Skin Irritation

Irritations, including conditions like eczema, can be tied back to your gut. The connection here is through the gut-skin axis, where a leaky gut allows particles to enter your bloodstream, causing inflammation and skin issues.

Allergies and Autoimmune Conditions

These can be worsened by poor gut health. When your gut flora is out of balance, it can lead to systemic inflammation, potentially triggering or aggravating these conditions.

Mood Issues and Migraines

These can be less obvious but equally important indicators of gut health. The gut-brain axis has an influence on this; neurotransmitters produced in the gut affect mental clarity and emotional well-being. An unhealthy gut can result in mood swings, anxiety, depression, and frequent headaches or migraines.

Signs of a "More Healthy" Gut

On the flip side, recognizing the signs of a healthy gut can provide immense relief and confidence in your overall well-being.

Healthy Bowel Movements

A healthy gut is characterized by regular, pain-free bowel movements that are well-formed and easy to pass. You should be able to have a bowel movement once a day or a few times a week without straining or discomfort. Your stools should be brown and hold their shape when flushed.

Constant Levels of Energy

You're also likely to experience a steady level of energy throughout the day without significant ebbs and flows when your gut is healthy. This indicates that your body is efficiently absorbing nutrients and not struggling with inflammation or other gut issues that could drain your energy levels. Sounds great, right?

Healthy Bowel Transit Time

Ideally, food should move through your digestive system at a steady pace—not too fast and not too slow. This is often called having a normal transit time (*Bowel Transit Time*, n.d.). With a healthy gut, you'll likely have a bowel movement once every 12–24 hours after eating a meal. If food moves too quickly, you may experience diarrhea or loose stools. If it moves too slowly, you may deal with constipation or feel sluggish after eating.

Normal Amounts of Gas and Bloating

Experiencing gas and bloating is normal, even with a healthy gut. However, excessive gas that causes significant discomfort or pain could be a sign of imbalance. With a healthy gut, you may experience mild bloating after a large meal, but it should subside within a couple of hours as your body digests the food properly. Frequent severe bloating that doesn't go away could point to issues like food intolerances, bacterial overgrowth, or other gut problems.

No Adverse Food Reactions

One of the key roles of the gut is to act as a barrier by preventing partially digested food particles or toxins from passing into your bloodstream. With a healthy, intact gut lining, you're less likely to experience negative reactions after eating foods. Symptoms like bloating, gas, diarrhea, rashes, fatigue, or brain fog after meals could signal a compromised gut lining that allows food particles to trigger an immune response in your body.

Mental Clarity and Stress Response

There is a strong gut-brain connection, so imbalances in your gut can impact your mental state. With a healthy gut, you're more likely to experience clear thinking, an ability to focus, and better resilience to stress. You'll feel more emotionally stable and less prone to mood swings or anxiety that could be linked to gut inflammation. Having a healthy gut supports optimal neurotransmitter production.

Gurgling Sounds in Your Stomach

Many people think the sounds your stomach makes always mean you're hungry. Dr. Pimentel, a medical and gut health professor, says these noises might mean your gut is shifting gears to clean itself like a dishwasher. The gurgling is due to something called the "migrating motor complex," which happens every 90 minutes between meals to clean your gut (Galloway, 2022). He explains that the gut works in two ways—eating and cleaning—similar to how a dishwasher operates. Giving the gut time to clean between meals is crucial for it to work well.

Causes of Poor Gut Health

There are many possible causes of poor gut health. Let's explore some of the main culprits.

Food Allergies and Sensitivities

When your body doesn't agree with certain foods, it can cause trouble in your gut. This happens when your body reacts badly to the food and causes swelling, which messes with your gut friends.

Imbalanced Diet

Eating too much junk food and not enough fibery stuff can make things go wrong in your gut. Your good gut buddies can become too hungry while the bad ones get too much food. This can cause a not-fun party in your tummy.

Chronic Stress

Being super stressed all the time can mess with your gut. This happens when your body gets ready to run from danger, but when there's no danger, it messes with your gut. The gut doesn't get as much blood when you're stressed, so things slow down.

Smoking

When you smoke, you're putting bad stuff into your body that can hurt your gut. This bad stuff can mess up the gut's protection and make the helpful bacteria go a little crazy. Smoking causes havoc in your gut.

Medications

Some medicines, especially antibiotics, can cause trouble in your gut. They don't just kick out the bad gut bacteria; they also kick out the good ones. This leaves your gut feeling a little empty and confused.

Medical Conditions

If you have irritable bowel syndrome (IBS) or celiac disease, your gut might not be feeling its best. IBS can make your gut uncomfortable, while celiac disease can upset your gut when you eat gluten. These conditions can really cause trouble with your gut.

Assessing Your Gut's Health

For a comprehensive assessment of your gut health, you might consider undergoing official tests conducted by medical professionals. Typically, these tests include stool analysis, breath tests, and blood tests. To proceed, you would consult with a healthcare provider who can recommend the best test based on your symptoms and health history. You can also consider trying an at-home test.

Here's what you can do to decide between at-home tests and professional tests:

- **Talk to a healthcare provider:** Always start by discussing your symptoms and concerns with a professional. They can guide you toward the most suitable testing method.
- **Evaluate the convenience:** At-home tests offer privacy and ease, requiring just a sample to be sent to a lab. Professional tests may require multiple visits but often provide more detailed insights.
- **Compare costs:** At-home tests can be more affordable, but check if your insurance covers professional testing.
- **Consider the accuracy:** While both methods can be effective, professional tests are often more comprehensive and tailored to your specific needs.

The differences and similarities between at-home tests and clinical tests are primarily in their scope and depth. At-home tests are more convenient and less invasive but may not offer the full range of diagnostics that a clinic can. Pros include ease and privacy, while cons may include less personalized guidance. Clinical tests, on the other hand, provide thorough and precise diagnostics under professional supervision but can be more time-consuming and expensive.

Where to Find At-Home Test Kits

- **Online retailers:** Websites for companies like Amazon, Walmart, and CVS often carry a variety of at-home gut health test kits.
- **Direct from manufacturers:** Companies such as Viome, Thryve, and Everlywell sell their test kits directly through their websites.

- **Local pharmacies:** Some larger pharmacy chains may stock basic gut health test kits.

Popular Types of At-Home Gut Health Tests

- **Microbiome tests:** Analyze the bacteria in your gut.
- **Food sensitivity tests:** Check for potential food intolerances.
- **Celiac disease tests:** Screen for gluten sensitivity.
- **H. pylori tests:** Detect the presence of Helicobacter pylori bacteria.

How to Use an At-Home Gut Health Test Kit

- **Read instructions carefully:** Each kit will have specific instructions.
- **Collect the sample:** This usually involves a stool sample or sometimes a blood spot or saliva.
- **Package the sample:** Follow the kit's guidelines for proper packaging.
- **Send to the lab:** Use the provided prepaid shipping label.
- **Wait for results:** Typically takes 2–4 weeks.
- **Interpret results:** Many companies provide online portals or detailed reports.

Things to Consider

- **FDA approval:** Check that the test is FDA-approved or cleared.
- **Privacy:** Understand the company's data privacy policies.
- **Follow up:** Consider discussing results with a healthcare professional.

- **Limitations:** At-home tests may not be as comprehensive as clinical tests.

While at-home tests can provide valuable insights, they should not replace professional medical advice or diagnosis.

Taking control of your digestive health, especially during menopause, can significantly enhance your quality of life. By understanding the signs of an unhealthy and healthy gut, knowing what causes gut issues, and considering both home-based and clinical tests, you can make informed decisions that empower you to achieve better health and well-being.

QUICK SELF-EVALUATION

Assessing your digestive health during menopause is crucial because it's a time of significant hormonal shifts that can impact many body systems, including your gut. To make this process both informative and engaging, I've put together a quiz to help you evaluate your digestive health. Think of it as a friendly conversation, one where we'll begin to uncover some valuable insights about your well-being.

First off, let's dive into the quiz. Grab a pen and paper or just mentally note your answers—whatever makes you feel most comfortable. This is a judgment-free zone!

Quiz: How's Your Gut Feeling Lately?

1. **How frequently do you feel gassy or bloated?**
   A. Rarely
   B. Occasionally
   C. Frequently
   D. Almost always

2. **Do you struggle with constipation or diarrhea?**
   A. Rarely
   B. Occasionally
   C. Frequently
   D. Almost always

3. **After meals, how often do you feel overly full or uncomfortable?**
   A. Rarely
   B. Occasionally
   C. Frequently
   D. Almost always

4. **How would you describe your energy levels?**
   A. High and consistent
   B. Typically good but sometimes low
   C. Often low and sluggish
   D. Mostly depleted and fatigued

5. **Do you notice any food sensitivities or intolerances?**
   A. Rarely or never
   B. A few
   C. Several
   D. Many

6. **What's your daily fiber intake like?**
   A. Adequate (25-30 grams): You are eating a large bowl of high-fiber cereal and a few servings of fruits, vegetables, and whole grains throughout the day.
   B. Fair (15–20 grams): You are eating a serving or two of high-fiber foods like beans, berries, or whole wheat bread.

C. Low (10–15 grams): You are eating mainly refined grains like pastries and white bread, meats, and low-fiber snacks.

D. Very low (<10 grams): You are mostly eating processed foods and refined carbohydrates like bread, rice, and cake.

7. **How are your stress levels?**
   A. Low
   B. Manageable
   C. High
   D. Overwhelming

8. **Do you take any probiotics or digestive aids?**
   A. Regularly
   B. Occasionally
   C. Rarely
   D. Never

Take a moment to tally up your responses, noting which letter you selected most frequently.

Here's what your answers may indicate:

- **Mostly As and Bs:** Your gut health seems to be in pretty good shape! Keep up with your current habits but stay attuned to any changes.
- **Mostly Cs:** There might be some aspects of your digestive health that need attention. Small changes can have a big impact.
- **Mostly Ds:** It's essential to address your digestive health more seriously. Consider consulting with a healthcare provider for tailored advice.

Understanding your results is just the beginning. It's vital to grasp why these questions matter, especially during menopause. Now that you've got a snapshot of your gut health, we will discuss in later chapters the practical steps you can take.

Your journey through menopause can be challenging, but taking control of your digestive health can make a significant difference. It's a blend of personal responsibility and acknowledging when you need a helping hand—whether that's reaching out to health-care professionals or simply recalibrating your lifestyle choices based on solid evidence and self-awareness.

Evaluating your gut health isn't just a box to check; it's an ongoing dialogue with your body. By staying informed and proactive, you're better equipped to navigate the ups and downs of menopause, ensuring that your overall well-being takes center stage. So take these insights to heart, and remember, it's all about finding balance while prioritizing your health above all else.

As we continue our exploration of the 7 **RESTORE Steps to Gut Health**, we now turn our focus to the effects of menopause on digestive health. In the next chapter, we will examine the impact it has on your GI tract and why.

2

EXAMINING THE EFFECT OF MENOPAUSE ON DIGESTIVE HEALTH

M arlene always thought she was fairly healthy. In her late 40s, she ate well, stayed active, and hardly had digestive problems. But as she neared her 50th birthday, she started noticing small changes in her body. It started with feeling bloated and uncomfortable after meals. She ignored it, thinking it was due to a tough week at work or a recipe that didn't turn out right.

These symptoms started to happen more often and got worse. Marlene began avoiding foods she used to enjoy, worried about how her stomach would react. Going out with friends made her anxious because she couldn't predict how her stomach would feel. She often felt too full and gassy, making her feel awkward and annoyed.

Marlene desperately wanted to figure out what was going on, so she asked her doctor for help. After some tests, the doctor said it might be related to her body changing because of menopause. Marlene was surprised she hadn't thought about menopause at all.

She began addressing her symptoms by adjusting her diet to incorporate more fiber and probiotics. She took up activities such as yoga and meditation to alleviate stress. She also became more attuned to her body's signals to steer clear of triggers that caused discomfort.

Menopause can be a confusing time with lots of unexpected changes. It can affect your emotions and your body, even impacting your digestion. Think of your stomach, which used to be reliable, now acting up and causing discomfort when you least expect it.

We started by considering the meaning of gut health, how it affects our overall well-being, and how to improve it. In this chapter, we'll dive into the second part of the 7 **RESTORE Steps to Gut Health**, which is all about **E**xamining the effect of menopause on digestive health. We will explore how menopause doesn't just change your hormones but can also disrupt your gut health.

Hormonal fluctuations during menopause do more than cause mood swings and hot flashes; they bring about substantial changes in your digestive system as well. For instance, declining levels of estrogen—a hormone known for its anti-inflammatory properties—can disturb the balance of bacteria in the gut. This imbalance often leads to uncomfortable symptoms such as bloating, constipation, and gas. Similarly, reduced estrogen levels can slow down the digestive process, affecting your overall gastrointestinal health. It's like navigating through a maze where each twist and turn presents new challenges to your once-straightforward path. Therefore, evaluating your digestive health in menopause isn't merely a task; it's a key aspect of managing this stage of life with confidence.

In this chapter, we'll investigate how menopause alters gut health and explore the interactions between your hormones and digestive system. You'll discover the impacts of decreased estrogen and progesterone levels on your gut microbiome and learn how these hormonal shifts create digestive issues.

We'll also discuss self-care strategies that can help manage these symptoms, offering practical advice on maintaining a balanced microbiome during this life-changing phase. By understanding these connections, you'll be better equipped to navigate the complexities of digestive health during menopause and make informed choices to support your well-being.

HOW MENOPAUSE AFFECTS GUT HEALTH

Menopause doesn't just impact your reproductive system—it also affects your gut health. The changes in the bacteria living in your gut during menopause can lead to digestive issues such as bloating, gas, and irregular bowel movements. These changes are influenced by hormonal shifts, particularly the decrease in estrogen levels. It's like having a party in your gut with disco music and funky bacteria dancing the night away! (Without your "parental" consent, of course.)

Bacteria at War With Your Declining Estrogen Levels

During menopause, the balance of bacteria in the gut shifts, influenced largely by the decline in estrogen levels. These hormonal changes can lead to a less diverse gut microbiome, which is often linked to various health issues. For many women, this means dealing with new and unexpected digestive symptoms. The gut, after all, isn't simply a food processing unit—it's a complex ecosystem that interacts with nearly every aspect of our health.

Research reveals that as estrogen diminishes, it can disrupt the harmonious community of gut bacteria, and in turn these bacteria also affect estrogen levels (Qi et al., 2021). This disruption may result in symptoms like bloating, gas, and irregular bowel movements. Interestingly, studies suggest that certain strains of beneficial bacteria decrease while harmful bacteria can increase, leading to an imbalance known as dysbiosis. Imagine your gut as a lush garden where the right mix of plants creates a healthy ecosystem. When menopause hits, it's like a sudden weather change that disrupts how these plants thrive and interact with each other.

Stormy Sea Inside the Digestive System

Our hormones control many body functions, including digestion. During menopause, It's like navigating a boat on a stormy sea—one small interference can cascade through the whole system, disrupting everything.

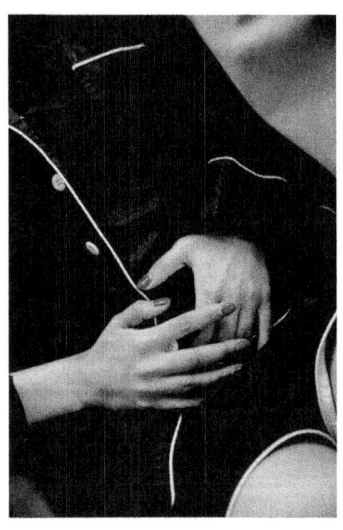

Estrogen helps keep the gut healthy by fighting inflammation. When estrogen levels decrease, this anti-inflammatory protection is reduced, leading to increased gut inflammation (Nie et al., 2018). Estrogen also helps regulate bile acid production. When estrogen levels drop, bile acid production can become impaired, which in turn slows down digestion (Phelps et al., 2019). The gut and hormones impact each other—they have what is known as a bidirectional relationship—causing a cycle of problems.

Lower estrogen and progesterone levels can slow down the movement of food through your digestive tract, leading to issues like constipation. On top of that, menopause often brings about a decrease in stomach acid production, which is vital for breaking down food and absorbing nutrients.

This hormonal tizzy can also affect the gut-brain axis, the communication network between the gut and brain. Stress and anxiety, which often accompany menopause due to hormonal changes, can further disturb digestive health. It's a bit of a domino effect; one piece falls out of place and the others quickly follow.

Changes in Estrogen Levels and Other Hormones

Estrogen isn't working alone here; progesterone, another key hormone that declines during menopause, plays a significant role in gut health. Progesterone tends to have a relaxing effect on the muscles of the digestive tract. As its levels drop, these muscles can become less efficient, contributing to issues like bloating and bowel irregularities.

The stress hormone cortisol can spike during menopause. Elevated cortisol levels can compromise gut health by increasing intestinal permeability, also called "leaky gut," where unwanted particles enter your bloodstream, prompting immune responses and inflammation.

Understanding and addressing these hormonal shifts can provide a clearer path to managing digestive health during menopause.

HOW SHIFTS IN HORMONE LEVELS AFFECT YOUR GUT'S WELL-BEING

We established in the previous section that our bodies are incredibly complex systems where hormone levels play a pivotal role in regulating various functions, including digestive processes. Estrogen and progesterone, the primary female hormones, fluctuate significantly during menopause and perimenopause, impacting your gut in numerous ways. High or low levels of these hormones can disturb the delicate balance of your GI system, leading to problems ranging from mild discomfort to severe distress.

Irritable Bowel Syndrome

Take, for instance, irritable bowel syndrome (IBS). Many women report the onset or worsening of IBS symptoms during menopause. The gut-brain axis—the communication network linking your central nervous system to your GI tract—depends heavily on hormonal signals. When estrogen levels drop, it can lead to increased sensitivity in the gut, meaning minor disruptions become exacerbated, causing pain and irregular bowel movements.

Here are some things you can do to manage IBS during this period:

- Maintain a detailed food and beverage log to help pinpoint potential triggers.
- Experiment with removing potential culprits from your diet one by one.
- Incorporate fiber-rich foods to aid digestion.
- Practice stress-relief techniques such as yoga or mindfulness meditation.

Issues With Abdominal Bloating

Bloating is another common symptom many women face due to hormonal fluctuations. Progesterone, which rises initially during perimenopause and falls precipitously as you reach menopause, can slow down your digestive process. This slowdown often leads to gas buildup and abdominal bloating, making you feel puffy and uncomfortable.

Here are some ways you can try to alleviate bloating:

- Eat smaller, more frequent meals instead of larger ones.
- Limit carbonated drinks and avoid chewing gum.
- Consider incorporating natural diuretics like cucumber or asparagus into your diet.

Diarrhea or Constipation

Issues with diarrhea or constipation can also pop up. Both conditions can be attributed to erratic hormone levels disrupting the fluid balance in your intestines.

Here are some ways you can manage these symptoms:

- Stay hydrated.
- Include probiotics like yogurt or fermented foods in your diet.
- Avoid high-fat and heavily fried foods.

Boosting Your Metabolism

Your metabolism is also not immune to these hormonal shifts. Menopause can slow down metabolic processes, making it harder to maintain an ideal weight and affecting how your body handles food.

Here are some ways you can try to boost your metabolism:

- Engage in regular physical activity, focusing on strength training.
- Opt for nutrient-dense foods.
- Get enough sleep.

Insufficient Nutrient Absorption

Nutrient absorption issues may also arise given that your digestive organs may not work as efficiently during this phase.

Here are some ways you can enhance nutrient absorption:

- Chew your food thoroughly.
- Consider supplements, but check with your healthcare provider first.
- Eat a well-balanced diet.

Leaky Gut Syndrome

Another concern is the integrity of the gut lining itself. Leaky gut syndrome, characterized by increased intestinal permeability, has been linked to fluctuating hormone levels.

Here are some ways to support gut integrity:

- Include collagen-rich foods or supplements in your diet.
- Reduce your intake of processed foods, sugar, and alcohol.
- Introduce bone broth or fermentable fibers.

Food Allergies and Intolerances

The onset of food allergies and intolerances can catch many women off guard.

Here are some things you can try if you suspect new food sensitivities:

- Start keeping a detailed food journal.

- Work with a nutritionist or healthcare provider to conduct an elimination diet.
- Gradually incorporate anti-inflammatory foods into your diet.

THE GUT-HORMONE CONNECTION

It's evident that gut health is interwoven with our hormone levels. An unhealthy gut microbiome can lead to hormonal imbalances, particularly affecting women during menopause. When your gut isn't functioning optimally, it can interfere with the body's ability to regulate hormones like estrogen. This imbalance can result in symptoms like weight gain, hot flashes, and mood swings becoming more pronounced.

Maintaining a healthy gut is crucial for overall well-being, especially during times of hormonal fluctuations. If you're experiencing any digestive issues or concerns, don't hesitate to reach out to your healthcare provider for guidance and support.

Realign Your Gut to Manage Menopause

Addressing gut health doesn't have to be overwhelming. It's about making small but meaningful changes. Incorporating a diet rich in fiber, for example, can promote healthy bowel movements and reduce constipation. Whole grains, fruits, vegetables, beans, and nuts are all excellent sources of dietary fiber. They help fuel the beneficial bacteria in your gut, allowing them to thrive and outcompete the harmful bacteria.

Drinking plenty of water aids digestion and helps maintain regular bowel movements. Dehydration can lead to constipation, which can make bloating and discomfort worse, so keep a glass of water handy throughout the day and make sure you're sipping regularly.

Good gut health can serve as a cornerstone for managing menopause more comfortably. When your digestive system is functioning optimally, it creates a foundation for better overall health. Symptoms like fatigue, brain fog, and even joint pain can be lessened by addressing gut health. Balancing your gut flora can boost nutrient absorption, ensuring your body gets the vital vitamins and minerals it needs during this transitional period.

A HOLISTIC APPROACH TO GUT HEALTH AND MENOPAUSE MANAGEMENT

As we explore the connections between menopause and gut health, it becomes evident that this relationship is not just beneficial but necessary for a smoother midlife journey. Hormonal shifts during menopause naturally disrupt the equilibrium within our bodies, and our guts are no exception. However, taking proactive steps toward nurturing your digestive health can transform your experience.

Incorporating more fermented foods into your diet can support gut diversity. Fermented foods contain natural probiotics, which, as we've already touched on, are beneficial for maintaining a healthy gut microbiome. Some options include kimchi, tempeh, and kombucha. Consuming these regularly can help repopulate your gut with beneficial bacteria, aiding in better digestion and overall well-being.

Another aspect to consider is the role of prebiotics—the food for your friendly gut bacteria. Prebiotics are found in foods like garlic, onions, leeks, asparagus, and bananas. Including these in your meals can support the growth of beneficial bacteria.

Physical activity is another powerful ally for both gut health and menopause management. Regular exercise can promote better digestion and enhance the motility of the gastrointestinal tract, reducing the risk of constipation. Activities like walking, yoga, and swimming not only offer physical benefits but also help in stress reduction—a crucial factor during menopause.

Sleep is equally important. Poor sleep patterns can negatively impact gut health, leading to an imbalance in the gut microbiota. Establishing a consistent sleep routine, practicing good sleep hygiene, and creating a restful environment can support both gut health and overall well-being during menopause.

When considering the interplay between menopause and gut health, it's crucial to listen to your body. Pay attention to how different foods and lifestyle choices affect your digestive system and overall health. Keeping a food diary can help you identify triggers or patterns and allow you to make informed adjustments.

The connection between gut health and menopause highlights the importance of viewing our health holistically. Every part of our body is interconnected, and nurturing one aspect often leads to positive ripple effects throughout. By focusing on gut health, you are investing in your long-term well-being, making the transition through menopause smoother and more manageable.

Embracing this holistic approach empowers you with control over your health. It emphasizes personal responsibility while acknowledging the need for supportive measures during challenging times. The evidence speaks for itself: A healthy gut can be a game-changer in your menopausal journey. It's time to give your gut the attention it deserves to foster a healthier, happier, and more balanced life.

PERSONALIZED WELLNESS WORKSHEET

While it's important to acknowledge the challenges presented by gut health in menopause, it's just as important to focus on what we can do about it. I firmly believe in putting the power back into your hands; understanding and managing these symptoms is well within your reach. Let's get started on setting some realistic goals to improve your digestive health during this life phase.

Creating a personalized worksheet can go a long way in helping you manage your digestive health. This will give you a structured approach and make it easier to track your progress. In the following sections, we'll look at some steps to help you along the way.

Identify Specific Goals

The first step in improving digestive health during menopause is to identify specific goals. This could be anything from reducing bloating to ensuring regular bowel movements. Make sure these goals are tailored to your personal experiences and needs. A good starting point could be

- increasing fiber intake.
- drinking more water.
- reducing processed food consumption.
- working exercise into your daily routine.

Assess Your Current Lifestyle

Before you can set realistic goals, evaluate where you currently stand. Note down your daily routine, dietary habits, and any symptoms you regularly experience. This self-assessment will serve as a baseline for measuring your progress. If you realize you're drinking only two glasses of water a day, you'll know it's something you need to work on.

Create a Daily Log

One effective way to keep track of your digestive health is by creating a daily log. Write down everything you eat and drink, noting how different foods affect your digestive system. Record your physical activity and stress levels as well. Stress can significantly impact gut health, so it's worth paying attention to.

Consider using a simple format like this:

- Date
- Meals (breakfast, lunch, dinner, and snacks)
- Water intake
- Physical activity
- Digestive symptoms (bloating, constipation, etc.)
- Stress levels and emotional state

Set Short-Term Goals

Setting smaller short-term goals can make the entire process feel less overwhelming. Short-term goals also offer the advantage of quick wins, which can be incredibly motivating. Here are some examples:

- This week, aim to drink 3 extra glasses of water each day.
- Try incorporating a 15-minute walk after meals.
- Add 1 serving of fruits or vegetables to every meal.

Track Your Progress

As you implement changes, use your daily log to track your progress. Regularly assessing this information allows you to make necessary adjustments. Perhaps you've noticed that eating certain foods exacerbates your symptoms; you can then decide to eliminate or reduce these from your diet.

Adjust When Necessary

Nobody's perfect, and it's important to remember that setbacks happen. If you find certain goals too challenging, don't hesitate to adjust them. The key is to continue moving forward, even if you're taking smaller steps than initially planned. Adaptability is crucial here; life's complexities sometimes mean that what works today might need tweaking tomorrow.

Consult Healthcare Providers

Always consult with your healthcare provider when setting more complex goals or making significant lifestyle changes. Their expertise can provide valuable insights that general advice cannot. They can also help ensure your new goals align with your health needs.

Make Use of Support Systems

It helps to have someone else involved in your journey. Whether it's a family member, a friend, or a professional, having someone to share your progress with can offer additional motivation.

Goal-setting is an ongoing process. Revisit and revise your goals periodically to reflect your progress and changing needs. Make a big deal about your achievements, even if they're small. Recognizing your efforts plays a critical role in maintaining momentum and staying motivated.

Quick Recap on the Process

Let's review what you need to do:

- **Goal setting:**
  - List specific goals related to your digestive health.
  - Include reasons why achieving these goals matters to you.
- **Daily log:**
  - Daily entries for meals and snacks, water intake, physical activity, digestive symptoms, and stress levels.
- **Short-term goals:**
  - Write down weekly targets.
  - Track your progress.
  - Mark completed tasks or achieved goals.
  - Summarize weekly or monthly progress.
  - Make notes on what worked, what didn't, and what needs adjustment.

Break the process down into easier-to-manage steps to help support your digestive health during menopause. Remember, it's important to find a balance. It's fine to put people before money and to rely on yourself and your community for support. We're all going through life's different stages together, staying strong and resilient.

I hope this guideline provides a solid foundation for improving your digestive health. Take it one step at a time, and don't forget to be kind to yourself throughout the journey.

As you steer through menopause, it's also a period of re-evaluation. It's an opportunity to adopt new lifestyle choices that support hormonal and digestive health. Every choice is a step toward nurturing your body through this change.

You are not alone. Many women share these experiences, and taking informed, mindful action can lead to thriving through menopause. It's about harmonizing with your body's changes, embracing every phase compassionately, and knowing that better days are ahead.

This book aims to provide you with practical advice you can implement immediately. In the next chapter, we will explore ways to strengthen your gut microbiome.

3

STRENGTHENING YOUR GUT MICROBIOME

I n her younger years, Lea could indulge in all her favorite foods —pizza, spicy curries, chocolate, even cake—without conse- quences. Her body seemed to handle it all with ease, with no weight gain or health issues in sight. But at 47, as perimenopause gradually started to move over to menopause, her gut started sending her new signals.

One day, she'd be doubled over with cramps. The next, she'd battle reflux or diarrhea, her once-predictable bathroom routine out of sync. And then there was the belly fat that crept up on her, stub- bornly sticking around no matter how active she was.

Despite following her doctor's advice—cutting calories, swapping sugar for zero-calorie alternatives, going low-carb—the changes just weren't happening. Lea felt like she was fighting her own body.

Her story is a familiar one. Many women going through menopause find themselves navigating dramatic gut health shifts tied to the fluctuating ovarian hormone levels of estrogen and progesterone. What once felt like second nature—making food choices based on cravings or calorie count—no longer applies.

These days, Lea is learning to listen to her gut's needs instead of her cravings. She's feeding her microbiome, that teeming community of bacteria living inside her, to support her overall well-being through this transition. It's an intimate new journey of tuning in to her body's signals and adapting as nature intends.

While the road hasn't been easy, Lea is coming to understand that good gut health is about more than just avoiding discomfort; it's about regaining balance, embracing change, and nurturing herself —body and microbes together—through menopause.

When your internal gut community becomes imbalanced, the effects can ripple throughout your body in surprising ways. In this chapter, we'll explore the third part of the 7 **RESTORE Steps to Gut Health**, which is all about **S**trengthening your gut microbiome.

You will learn how dietary choices, lifestyle changes, and additional strategies can nurture a healthy gut microbiome, alleviating some of these challenging symptoms. From incorporating fiber-rich foods to leveraging the benefits of fermented goodies, we'll explore practical steps to fortify your inner ecosystem. Get ready to discover how small adjustments improve your gut health and overall well-being.

By understanding and caring for our gut health, especially during critical times like menopause, we take control of a fundamental part of our well-being. Embracing this proactive approach can yield long-lasting benefits, empowering us to lead healthier, more vibrant lives.

THE ROLE OF GUT BACTERIA IN HEALTH AND HORMONAL BALANCE

Let's build on what we discussed in Chapters 1 and 2. The human body is home to trillions of microorganisms, with the majority residing in our digestive tract. The complex ecosystem called the gut microbiome is vital for supporting our overall health as it affects aspects such as digestion, immunity, mood, and hormonal regulation.

An intricate relationship exists between gut bacteria and various aspects of human health, such as hormonal regulation. This is particularly relevant for women approaching or experiencing menopause as hormonal changes during this period can significantly impact gut health and vice versa.

Understanding Gut Bacteria and the Microbiome

The gut microbiome plays an important role in

- digesting food.
- producing vitamins (like B and K).
- protecting against harmful bacteria.
- regulating the immune system.
- influencing metabolism and hormone production.

Gut Bacteria and Common Health Conditions

Research has shown associations between gut bacteria imbalances and various health conditions. According to a comprehensive review published in the *New England Journal of Medicine*, "The gut microbiome has been implicated in a wide range of human disorders, including inflammatory bowel disease, cardiovascular disease, metabolic diseases, and cancer" (Lynch & Pedersen, 2016).

This research supports the associations we'll discuss in the following sections.

Obesity, Type 2 Diabetes, Kidney Disease, and Heart Disease

- Certain gut bacteria may contribute to inflammation and metabolic disorders.
- Imbalances in your gut bacteria can affect how your body processes and stores energy from food.

Inflammatory Bowel Disease

- Crohn's disease and ulcerative colitis are associated with less diverse gut microbiomes.
- Certain bacteria may trigger or exacerbate inflammation in the gut.

Colon Cancer

- Some gut bacteria produce compounds that may promote colon cancer.
- A diverse, healthy microbiome may help protect against colon cancer.

Mental Health and Neurological Conditions

- The gut-brain axis links gut health to mental health.
- Imbalances in gut bacteria have been associated with anxiety, depression, and autism.

Arthritis

Arthritis is a chronic condition characterized by inflammation in the joints, leading to pain and stiffness that can impact daily life.

- Research has revealed an intriguing link between gut health and joint inflammation, suggesting that certain gut bacteria may play an important role in triggering or exacerbating the condition (Jeyaraman et al., 2023).
- Maintaining a healthy gut microbiome appears to offer protective benefits, potentially reducing systemic inflammation and alleviating symptoms for those affected by arthritis. Understanding this connection opens new avenues for treatment and prevention, highlighting the important interplay between our digestive health and overall wellness.

Gut Health During Menopause and Perimenopause

Maintaining a healthy gut microbiome is particularly important during menopause and perimenopause due to

- hormonal fluctuations affecting gut function.
- increased risk of certain health conditions.
- potential impact on menopausal symptoms.

The Link Between Gut Bacteria and Hormones

An unhealthy gut microbiome can contribute to

- estrogen imbalances.
- thyroid dysfunction.
- cortisol irregularities.

Research Findings

Recent studies have provided evidence for the gut-hormone connection, which we'll explore in the following sections.

Study on Gut Microbiome and Sex Hormone-Related Diseases

- Links between gut bacteria and conditions like polycystic ovary syndrome and endometriosis were found.
- Suggests the potential for microbiome-based treatments for hormonal disorders.
- "The bidirectional relationship between the gut microbiome and circulating estrogen levels suggests that the gut microbiome may influence the risk of developing estrogen-related diseases" (Baker et al., 2017).

Study on Menopausal Syndrome and Gut Microbes

- Showed differences in gut microbiome composition between pre- and postmenopausal women.
- Certain bacteria were associated with the severity of menopausal symptoms.
- "The abundance of Firmicutes was significantly higher in the intestine of postmenopausal women... [and] the severity of menopausal syndrome was positively correlated with the abundance of Firmicutes" (Liu et al., 2022).

These findings support the idea of maintaining a healthy gut microbiome, especially during menopause.

HOW TO CULTIVATE A HEALTHY GUT MICROBIOME

Fiber is an essential element in maintaining a healthy relationship between gut bacteria and hormones. Let's explore how a fiber-rich diet can nourish beneficial gut bacteria and promote a balanced microbiome.

The Role of Fiber

Fiber acts as a prebiotic, which is food for your good gut bacteria, fostering an environment where they can thrive and in turn support optimal hormone regulation.

Fiber feeds beneficial gut bacteria. These bacteria produce short-chain fatty acids that can

- reduce inflammation.
- support hormone balance.
- improve insulin sensitivity.

Nurturing Your Gut Microbiome

To support a healthy gut biome, incorporate fermented foods like yogurt, kefir, and sauerkraut in your diet. These foods are packed with probiotics, the beneficial bacteria that can replenish your gut. Commit to a diet high in fiber obtained from fruits, vegetables, whole grains, and legumes to ensure that your gut bacteria remain well-fed and robust.

Avoid excessive use of antibiotics unless necessary as they can wipe out beneficial bacteria along with harmful ones. Reducing stress through mindfulness practices like yoga and meditation can also benefit your gut health by promoting a more stable and harmonious internal ecosystem.

Probiotic Supplements

When selecting probiotics for gut health, look for supplements containing Lactobacillus and Bifidobacterium strains, which have been extensively studied and are known to help with various digestive issues. Safe and effective usage involves reading the product instructions carefully and following the recommended dosage.

Probiotics can take some time to show results, typically a few days to several weeks. Be mindful of potential side effects, such as gas, bloating, or an upset stomach, especially when you first start taking them. Start with a lower dose and gradually increase it to mitigate these side effects.

Choosing Probiotic Supplements

When shopping for probiotic supplements, it's important to understand colony-forming units (CFUs) and other factors that affect quality and efficacy. The information in the following sections serves as a guide post to help you make the right choice about supplements that may work for you.

Learning About CFUs

CFUs indicate the number of feasible bacteria in a probiotic supplement (*Probiotic Supplements Dosage*, 2019):

- **Typical CFU ranges:** Most probiotic supplements contain between 1 billion and 100 billion CFUs per dose.
- **General guideline:** For general health maintenance, supplements with 1 to 10 billion CFUs are often sufficient.

- **Higher CFU counts:** For specific health conditions, your healthcare provider might recommend higher doses, sometimes up to 100 billion CFUs or more.

Shopping Guidelines

- **Check CFU count:** Look for products that specify the CFU count at the end of the product's shelf life, not at the time of manufacture.
- **Strain diversity:** Choose products with multiple strains of bacteria as different strains can have different benefits.
- **Research-backed strains:** Look for well-studied strains like Lactobacillus acidophilus, Bifidobacterium longum, or Lactobacillus rhamnosus GG.
- **Storage requirements:** Some probiotics require refrigeration to maintain potency. Check the label for storage instructions.
- **Packaging:** Choose products in dark opaque bottles that protect the bacteria from light and moisture.
- **Expiration date:** Always check and adhere to the expiration date.
- **Delivery method:** Some probiotics use special coatings or technologies to ensure the bacteria survive stomach acid.
- **Prebiotics:** Some products include prebiotics, which are "food" for the probiotic bacteria and can enhance their effectiveness.

Examples of CFU Counts for Different Purposes

The following daily CFU counts are typically used for different purposes (Ouwehand, 2017):

- **General health maintenance:** 10–20 billion CFUs
- **Antibiotic-associated diarrhea prevention:** 10–20 billion CFUs
- **IBS symptom management:** 20–50 billion CFUs
- **Specific therapeutic uses:** 50–100+ billion CFUs (under medical supervision)

More CFUs don't always mean better results. The right probiotic and dose can vary based on your specific needs and health conditions. It's always best to consult with a healthcare provider for personalized advice.

Probiotics for Hormonal Balance

For hormonal balance, probiotic strains can offer targeted benefits. Supplements designed for hormone regulation often include Lactobacillus and Bifidobacterium species, which have been linked to improved vaginal health, reduced risk of urinary tract infections, and reduced inflammation.

Another beneficial option is Bacillus species, which are spore-forming bacteria that can survive the digestive system better than some other strains, ensuring they reach the intestines where they can be most effective.

When choosing probiotics for hormone health, ensure the product lists the specific strains it contains along with a sufficient CFU count. The ingredients should be free of unnecessary additives or fillers, and usage instructions should be followed closely.

A Holistic Dietary Approach

Keeping a healthy gut microbiome involves a holistic approach that includes dietary adjustments, lifestyle changes, and potentially incorporating probiotic supplements. By cutting out sugar and processed foods, reducing red meat consumption, getting adequate sleep, and incorporating regular exercise, you create an environment that supports a thriving gut.

With intentional choices and informed actions, achieving a balanced gut microbiome is entirely within reach, paving the way for improved overall health. While self-care and dietary habits are pivotal, consulting healthcare professionals for personalized advice can provide another layer of assurance in your journey toward a healthier gut and, consequently, a healthier you.

FOODS FOR GOOD DIGESTIVE HEALTH

Supporting what we discussed in the previous section, the microbiome diet focuses on nurturing the trillions of bacterial inhabitants residing in your digestive tract. These beneficial microorganisms are pivotal for breaking down food, producing vitamins, and maintaining overall health. The diet focuses on eating a variety of foods that are high in fiber, fermented, and whole to support a healthy balance of gut bacteria. By doing so, we can enhance our digestion, reduce inflammation, and potentially ease some menopausal symptoms.

Yogurt

Yogurt, especially those marked as having live cultures, has good bacteria that help keep your stomach healthy. It's a versatile food that can be enjoyed at breakfast or as a snack. When choosing yogurt, opt for plain varieties to avoid added sugars, which can disrupt the gut's delicate balance.

Kefir

Kefir is another powerhouse in the world of fermented foods. This tangy dairy drink is loaded with probiotics, even more than yogurt. It aids in promoting a healthy bacterial balance, which is essential for a well-functioning digestive system. Regular consumption of kefir can help improve lactose digestion, which can be particularly useful during menopause when digestive sensitivities might increase.

Kombucha

Kombucha is a fermented tea that contains a mix of probiotics and enzymes, supporting gut health and digestion. Drinking kombucha regularly can introduce beneficial bacteria into your digestive system. Choose varieties with low sugar content to maximize gut health benefits.

Makgeolli

Makgeolli is a traditional Korean rice wine made from fermented rice. It offers a unique sweet and slightly tangy flavor. Due to its fermentation process, it is rich in probiotics, which promote gut health by aiding digestion and supporting a balanced gut microbiome. It also contains vitamins B and C and dietary fiber, contributing to overall wellness. Consume moderately as it contains alcohol.

Miso

Miso is a soybean paste that contains good bacteria for your gut. It's a staple in Japanese cuisine and can be used to make soups, marinades, or dressings. Its probiotic content helps improve digestion and supports the gut microbiome.

Natto

Natto, a fermented soybean product, is rich in probiotics and vitamin K2. Its unique flavor might take some getting used to, but it significantly benefits gut health and bone density. Try natto with rice or added to salads for a gut-boosting meal.

Kimchi

Kimchi is a spicy Korean dish made from pickled vegetables and contains healthy bacteria. It offers similar benefits to sauerkraut, enhancing gut health and digestion. Enjoy kimchi as a side dish or incorporate it into stir-fries and sandwiches.

Sauerkraut

Sauerkraut, a type of fermented cabbage, is rich in probiotics—beneficial bacteria that can enhance gut health. These microorganisms assist in balancing the gut microbiome, reducing bloating, and improving intestinal health. Incorporating sauerkraut into your meals can be as simple as adding a small side serving to your main dish.

Tempeh

Tempeh, a fermented soy product, is rich in probiotics and protein. It helps create a varied and healthy collection of gut bacteria. Use tempeh as a meat substitute in stir-fries, salads, or sandwiches.

Phytoestrogen-Rich Foods

Foods like soy, flaxseeds, and tofu mimic estrogen in the body, potentially easing some menopausal symptoms related to lower estrogen levels.

Almonds

Almonds are rich in prebiotics, which are types of fiber that help good bacteria in the gut. They also offer vitamin E and healthy fats, contributing to overall well-being. A handful of almonds can make for a perfect snack, promoting both gut health and hormonal balance.

Lentils

Lentils are fiber-rich legumes that support a healthy digestive system. They provide prebiotics to nourish your gut bacteria and contain protein, making them an excellent addition to a balanced diet. Adding lentils to soups, stews, or salads can help keep your gut flora thriving.

Whole Grains

Whole grains like oats, brown rice, and barley offer soluble and insoluble fibers that keep the digestive system moving smoothly. These grains behave like prebiotics in your gut by feeding the good bacteria. Eat different whole grains to keep your gut healthy.

Salmon

Salmon is high in omega-3 fatty acids, which reduce inflammation in the body. Omega-3s help keep the gut lining strong and support healthy digestion. Regularly incorporating salmon into your diet can provide these essential nutrients.

Apples

Apples have a lot of soluble fiber, especially pectin, which helps good bacteria in the gut grow. This contributes to better digestion. Enjoy apples whole, sliced, or blended into smoothies to reap their gut-friendly benefits.

Papaya

Papaya consists of a natural enzyme called papain that helps break down proteins and aids digestion. Eating fresh papaya or drinking its juice can support a healthy digestive system.

Beets

Beets are high in fiber and antioxidants, supporting liver detoxification and digestive health. Roasted, boiled, or juiced beets can easily become part of your diet to promote a healthy gut environment.

Dark Green Vegetables

Dark green vegetables like spinach, kale, and broccoli are high in fiber and nutrients that fuel a healthy gut microbiome. Their fiber content aids in regular bowel movements and feeds beneficial gut bacteria. Incorporate these greens into your meals daily.

Bone Broth

Bone broth is rich in gelatin, which aids in curing and sealing the gut lining. It is packed with nutrients that promote general health. Enjoy warm bone broth by sipping it or using it as a foundation for your soups and stews.

Gluten-Free Foods

For some women, gluten can exacerbate digestive issues. Opting for gluten-free grains like quinoa, rice, and millet can alleviate discomfort and support a healthier digestive system. Ensuring a varied diet is key, so experiment with different gluten-free options to sustain gut health.

Apple Cider Vinegar

Apple cider vinegar is renowned for its potential digestive benefits. It helps maintain an acidic environment in the stomach, which is crucial for proper digestion. You can incorporate apple cider vinegar into your diet by mixing a tablespoon with water before meals or using it as a salad dressing base.

Chia Seeds

Filled with nutrients and high in fiber, chia seeds, when soaked, form a gel-like consistency that helps support digestive health by promoting regular bowel movements. Add chia seeds to yogurt, oatmeal, smoothies, or drinks.

Fennel

Fennel has been traditionally used to ease digestive discomfort. It contains compounds that can relax the digestive tract and alleviate bloating. Add fennel to your meals or steep it in hot water to create a soothing digestive tea.

Ginger

Ginger has long been known for its digestive benefits. It can help lessen swelling and calm the stomach. Adding fresh ginger to teas, smoothies, or meals can aid in digestion and provide relief from nausea.

Peppermint

Peppermint has soothing properties that can relieve digestive upset. Drinking peppermint tea or adding fresh peppermint leaves to dishes can provide calming effects on the digestive system.

By mindfully incorporating these foods into your diet, you can cultivate a healthier gut microbiome, which in turn may help you manage your menopause symptoms. It's about finding what works best for you and creating sustainable habits that prioritize both your health and pleasure in eating.

RECIPES FOR A HEALTHY GUT MICROBIOME

Let's get to know the wonderful world of gut-friendly recipes, shall we? Cultivating a healthy gut microbiome is more than just a trend; it's integral to overall well-being, particularly for women navigating menopause and associated digestive health issues. To help you support your gut health, I've compiled some easy and delicious recipes for breakfast, lunch, dinner, dessert, and snacks that balance the use of cost-effective ingredients with substantial nutritional benefits.

Breakfast Recipes

Start your morning by fueling your body the right way.

Recipe 1: Gut-Healing Smoothie Bowl

Ingredients & tools

- 1/2 cup plain yogurt
- 1 tbsp chia seeds
- 1/2 cup spinach
- 1 banana
- 1 tbsp almond butter
- 1/2 cup unsweetened almond milk
- Some ice cubes
- Blender, bowl, and spoon

Instructions

- Mix all ingredients until smooth.
- Serve topped with fresh berries in a bowl.

Why this is good for your gut

Packed with probiotics from the yogurt and fiber from chia seeds and spinach, this smoothie bowl helps maintain a balanced gut flora.

Recipe 2: Oatmeal with Flaxseeds and Berries

Ingredients & tools

- 1 cup rolled oats
- 2 cups water
- 1 tbsp ground flaxseeds
- 1/2 cup mixed berries
- 1 tsp honey
- Pot, spoon, and bowl

Instructions

- Cook oats in water until soft.
- Stir in flaxseeds, then top with berries and honey.
- For overnight oats, prepare them in a glass container the prior evening and warm them up for breakfast.

Why this is good for your gut

Oats are rich in soluble fiber, which supports beneficial bacteria. Flaxseeds add omega-3 fatty acids and fiber, enhancing anti-inflammatory benefits.

Recipe 3: Avocado Toast with Sauerkraut

Ingredients & tools

- 1 slice whole grain bread
- 1/2 avocado
- 1 tbsp sauerkraut
- Salt and pepper to taste
- Toaster, fork, knife, and plate

Instructions

- Toast the bread to your desired level.
- Mash the avocado onto the toast and top with sauerkraut.
- Season with salt and pepper.

Why this is good for your gut

Avocado offers healthy fats, while sauerkraut brings probiotics to the table.

Recipe 4: Chia Seed Pudding

Ingredients & tools

- 3 tbsp chia seeds
- 1 cup coconut milk
- 1 tbsp maple syrup
- 1 tbsp collagen peptides
- Jar with lid and spoon

Instructions

- Combine all ingredients in a jar and stir well.
- Refrigerate overnight.

Why this is good for your gut

Chia seeds expand in liquid and form a gel-like consistency, which aids digestion and ensures prolonged gut health benefits. Collagen supports a healthy microbiome, which plays a vital role in digestion and overall health.

Recipe 5: Kefir Parfait

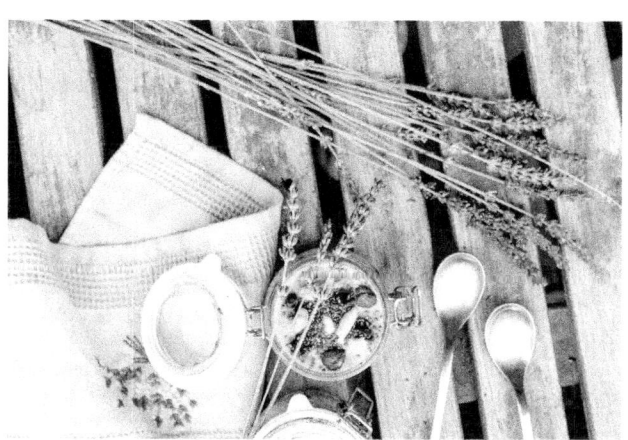

Ingredients & tools

- 1 cup kefir
- 1/2 cup granola
- 1/2 cup berries
- Some nuts for garnish (optional)
- Glass and spoon

Instructions

- Layer the kefir, granola, and berries in a glass. Sprinkle on remaining berries, granola, and some nuts if desired.

Why this is good for your gut

Kefir is a probiotic powerhouse that promotes good gut bacteria, and granola adds prebiotic fibers.

Lunch Recipes

Boost your gut health with these delicious and nutritious lunch recipes!

Recipe 6: Quinoa Salad with Vegetables

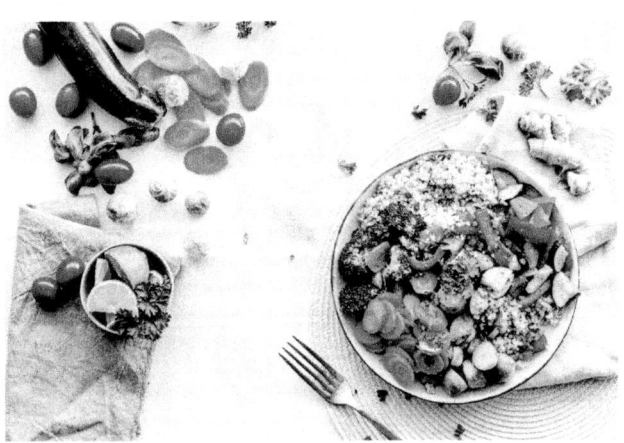

Ingredients & tools

- 1 cup cooked quinoa
- 1/2 cup vegetables (preferably fermented)
- 1 tbsp olive oil

- Juice of half a lemon
- Mixing bowl, fork, and spoon

Instructions

- Mix all ingredients in a bowl and serve.

Why this is good for your gut

Quinoa provides fiber and protein; fermented veggies add beneficial bacteria.

Recipe 7: Chicken and Veggie Wrap

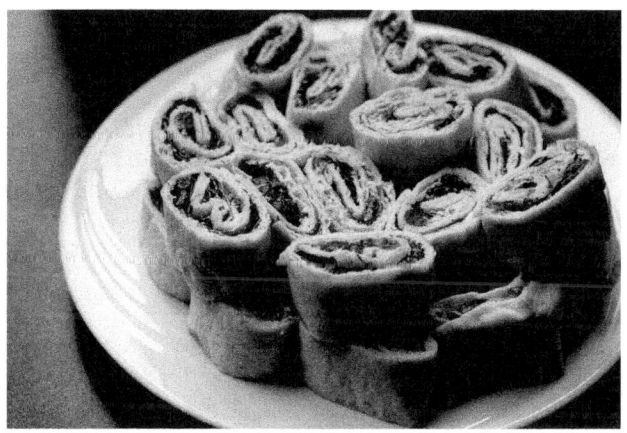

Ingredients & tools

- 1 whole grain wrap
- 1 grilled chicken breast
- 1 cup mixed greens
- 1/2 avocado
- 1 tbsp hummus
- Knife, cutting board, and plate

Instructions

- Spread hummus on the wrap.
- Add sliced chicken, mixed greens, and avocado.
- Roll up and cut in half.

Why this is good for your gut

This wrap includes fiber-rich greens and healthy fats from avocado.

Recipe 8: Miso Soup with Tofu and Wakame (Chen, 2024)

Ingredients & tools

- 4 cups water
- 2 tbsp miso paste
- 1 block tofu
- 1 tbsp dried wakame seaweed
- Pot, ladle, and bowls

Instructions

- Bring water to a boil, reduce heat, add cubed tofu and soaked wakame.
- Simmer gently for about 3 minutes or until heated through.
- Dilute miso paste with a spoon of soup, add to the pot, and stir to dissolve
- Ladle into bowls and serve hot.

Why this is good for your gut

Miso is fermented and contains live cultures that benefit gut health.

Recipe 9: Lentil and Beetroot Salad

Ingredients & tools

- 1 cup cooked lentils
- 1 roasted beetroot, diced
- 2 tbsp vinaigrette
- Mixing bowl and spoon

Instructions

- Combine lentils, beetroot, and vinaigrette in a bowl.
- Mix gently and serve.

Why this is good for your gut

Both lentils and beets are high in fiber, aiding in digestive health.

Recipe 10: Turmeric Chickpea Salad

Ingredients & tools

- 1 can chickpeas, drained
- 1 tbsp turmeric
- 2 tbsp olive oil
- 1 cup cucumber, diced
- Mixing bowl and spoon

Instructions

- Mix chickpeas with turmeric and olive oil.
- Add cucumber and toss everything together.

Why this is good for your gut

Turmeric has anti-inflammatory properties, and chickpeas provide prebiotics.

Dinner Recipes

Each of the following dinner recipes promises delightful flavors and caters to nurturing a healthy gut microbiome. Let's explore.

Recipe 11: Salmon With Asparagus and Garlic Yogurt Sauce

Ingredients & tools

- 2 salmon fillets
- 1 bunch asparagus
- 3 garlic cloves
- 1 cup plain yogurt (preferably Greek)
- 1 tbsp olive oil
- Baking sheet, oven, and mixing bowl

Instructions

- Preheat oven to 400 °F (200 °C).
- Place salmon and asparagus on a baking sheet and drizzle with olive oil.
- Bake for 15 minutes.
- Mix minced garlic into yogurt for sauce.

- Serve salmon and asparagus with a dollop of garlic yogurt sauce.

Why this is good for your gut

Salmon is rich in omega-3s, which aid gut inflammation, and Greek yogurt adds valuable probiotics.

Recipe 12: Vegetable Stir-Fry with Kimchi

Ingredients & tools

- 1 cup bell peppers, sliced
- 1 cup broccoli florets
- 1 cup peas
- 2 tbsp soy sauce
- 1/2 cup kimchi
- Wok, spatula, and plate

Instructions

- Sauté vegetables in a wok with olive oil until tender.
- Add soy sauce and toss well.
- Serve topped with kimchi.

Why this is good for your gut

The diversity of vegetables provides various fibers, and kimchi contains lactic acid bacteria.

Recipe 13: Spaghetti Squash with Marinara

Ingredients & tools

- 1 squash
- 2 cups marinara sauce
- 1 tbsp olive oil
- Salt and pepper to taste
- Baking dish, fork, knife, and saucepan

Instructions

- Cut squash in half and remove seeds.
- Drizzle cut squash halves with olive oil, season, and bake at 375 °F (190 °C) for 40 minutes.
- Scrape out squash strands with a fork.
- Heat marinara sauce in a saucepan and pour over squash strands.
- Place squash strands (spaghetti) back into the squash (using it as a bowl) or eat on a plate.

Why this is good for your gut

Spaghetti squash offers a low-calorie, fiber-rich alternative to pasta.

Recipe 14: Tempeh Tacos

Ingredients & tools

- 1 block tempeh
- 1 packet taco seasoning
- 8 small corn tortillas

- 1 cup shredded lettuce
- 1 avocado
- Salsa
- Frying pan and spoon

Instructions

- Crumble tempeh into a frying pan and cook with taco seasoning until heated.
- Assemble tacos with tempeh, lettuce, avocado slices, and salsa.

Why this is good for your gut

Tempeh adds plant-based proteins and probiotics.

Recipe 15: Butternut Squash Soup

Ingredients & tools

- 1 butternut squash
- 4 cups vegetable broth
- 1 onion
- 2 garlic cloves
- 1 tbsp olive oil
- Pot, blender, cutting board, and knife

Instructions

- Sauté chopped onion and garlic in olive oil until translucent.
- Add peeled, diced squash and broth. Simmer until the squash is tender.

- Blend until smooth.

Why this is good for your gut

This soup is loaded with vitamins and fiber, promoting digestion and gut health.

Dessert & Snack Recipes

Discover yummy good-for-you recipes that promote a happy, healthy gut while satisfying your sweet tooth!

Recipe 16: Yogurt and Berry Parfait

Ingredients & tools

- 1 cup plain yogurt (preferably Greek)
- 1/2 cup mixed berries
- 1 tbsp honey
- Glass and spoon

Instructions

- Layer yogurt, berries, and honey in a glass.
- Serve.

Why this is good for your gut

Greek yogurt's probiotics and fiber-rich berries make this parfait a perfect gut-friendly snack.

Recipe 17: Carrot and Ginger Muffins

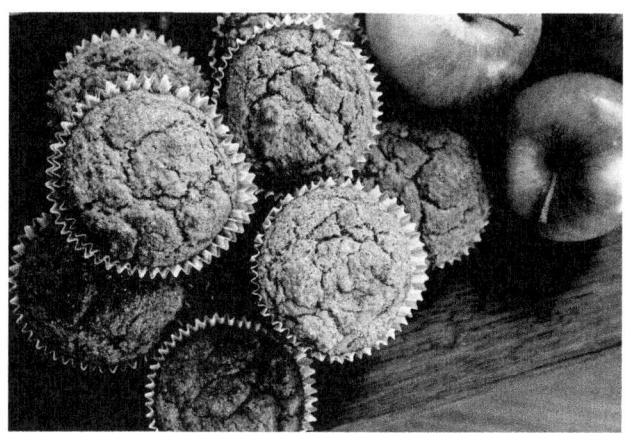

Ingredients & tools

- 2 cups finely grated carrots
- 1 cup whole wheat flour
- 1 cup all-purpose flour
- 2/3 cup olive oil
- 1 tsp ginger powder
- 3 large eggs
- 1 cup coconut sugar
- 1/2 tsp sea salt
- 2 tsp cinnamon powder
- 1 tsp vanilla
- 1-1/2 tsp baking soda
- Mixing bowl and spoon, muffin tin, and oven

Instructions

- Preheat oven to 375 °F (190 °C). Lightly grease muffin tin or use paper muffin cups.
- Mix all ingredients in a bowl.

- Spoon batter into muffin tins and bake for 15–20 minutes.

Why this is good for your gut

Carrots offer prebiotic fibers, ginger helps with digestion, and cinnamon helps gut bacteria thrive.

Recipe 18: Apple and Peanut Butter Slices

Ingredients & tools

- 1 apple
- 2 tbsp sugar-free peanut butter
- Knife and plate

Instructions

- Slice the apple.
- Spread peanut butter on each slice.

Why this is good for your gut

Apples contain pectin, a prebiotic fiber that feeds good bacteria.

Recipe 19: Frozen Banana Bites

Ingredients & tools

- 2 bananas
- 1/2 cup dark chocolate chips
- 1 tbsp coconut oil
- Microwave-safe bowl, parchment paper, and freezer

Instructions

- Melt chocolate chips with coconut oil in the microwave.
- Dip banana slices into the chocolate and place them on parchment paper.
- Freeze until solid.

Why this is good for your gut

Bananas are prebiotics that help fuel beneficial gut bacteria. Dark chocolate helps to grow good bacteria in the gut and eases issues like constipation and IBS.

Recipe 20: Almond Butter Energy Balls (Claudepierre, 2024)

Ingredients & tools

- 1 cup rolled oats
- 1/2 cup almond butter
- 1 tbsp chia seeds
- 1/4 cup honey
- Mixing bowl, spoon, and fridge

Instructions

- Mix all ingredients in a bowl.
- Refrigerate for 10–15 minutes.
- Lightly coat your hands with oil and dust them with flour to prevent sticking.
- Form into balls and refrigerate.
- Consume within a week or store in the freezer for up to 3 months. Thaw at room temperature.

Why this is good for your gut

These energy balls combine fiber, healthy fats, and chia seeds for an excellent source of nutrients for gut health.

5 Refreshing Drinks to Support Gut Health During Menopause

Looking for delicious ways to boost your gut health and potentially ease menopausal symptoms? These drink recipes offer a blend of refreshing flavors and beneficial ingredients.

Recipe 21: Probiotic Powerhouse Smoothie

Ingredients & tools

- 1 cup kefir
- 1 banana
- 1 tbsp honey (or a natural sweetener)
- 1 tbsp chia seeds
- Handful of spinach
- Blender, measuring cups, and spoons

Instructions

- Add kefir, banana, honey, chia seeds, and spinach to a blender.
- Blend until smooth.

Why this is good for your gut

Kefir and bananas contain beneficial bacteria that can help restore balance to your gut microbiome. Chia seeds provide fiber that promotes healthy digestion, and spinach is rich in antioxidants that can help protect your gut cells from damage.

Recipe 22: Antioxidant and Fiber Blast

Ingredients & tools

- 1 cup almond milk
- 1 cup mixed berries
- 1 cup spinach
- 1 tbsp flaxseeds
- Blender, measuring cups, and spoons

Instructions

- Add berries, spinach, almond milk, and flaxseeds to a blender.
- Blend until smooth.

Why this is good for your gut

Berries and spinach are rich in antioxidants, which can help protect your gut cells from damage. Almond milk contains fiber that supports improved digestion and prevents constipation. The high fiber content in flaxseeds has prebiotic properties that are beneficial for your gut health and hormone balance.

Recipe 23: Cooling and Hydrating Cucumber Mint Water

Ingredients & tools

- 1 cucumber, sliced
- Handful of fresh mint leaves
- 1 pitcher filled with water
- Lemon slices (optional)
- Pitcher and measuring cup

Instructions

- Combine cucumber, mint, water, and lemon slices in a pitcher.
- Chill in the refrigerator for a few hours.

Why this is good for your gut

Cucumber water keeps you hydrated, assists with weight loss, and is filled with antioxidants to help protect you against diseases. Cucumbers boost bone health as they contain lots of vitamin K.

Recipe 24: Plant-Based Soy Banana Protein Shake

Ingredients & tools

- 1 cup soy milk
- 1 banana
- 1 tbsp peanut butter
- Some ice cubes
- Measuring cups, spoons, and blender

Instructions

- Add soy milk, banana, peanut butter, and ice cubes to a blender.
- Blend until smooth.

Why this is good for your gut

This energizing combination can even be used as a post-workout smoothie. Protein shakes aid with muscle repair after exercise, boost your metabolism, and help with weight loss. Bananas improve your digestive health and moderate your blood sugar levels.

Recipe 25: Creamy Green Spinach Avo Smoothie

Ingredients & tools

- 1 cup spinach
- 1 cup coconut water
- 1 avocado
- Juice of 1 lime
- Blender, measuring cups, and spoons

Instructions

- Add avocado, spinach, coconut water, and lime juice to a blender.
- Blend until creamy.

Why this is good for your gut

The healthy fats in avocados help support hormonal balance during menopause, and the fiber in avocados and spinach promotes a healthy gut microbiome. This smoothie provides essential vitamins and minerals like iron, calcium, and vitamin K. Coconut water is hydrating, which helps with digestion and can relieve menopausal symptoms.

These recipes utilize readily available ingredients known to support gut health and potentially alleviate some menopausal symptoms. They are easy to prepare and taste delicious, too. Incorporating foods rich in fiber, probiotics, and anti-inflammatory properties into your daily diet helps you take significant steps toward better digestive health. The journey to gut health is continuous, and mealtime is an opportunity to support your body's well-being. Enjoy cooking, eating, and feeling great!

As you move forward, consider making intentional choices that support your gut microbiome. Welcome the journey toward a balanced gut, knowing each step brings you closer to enhanced overall health and harmony. After all, caring for your gut is caring for your entire body.

In Chapter 4, we'll look even deeper into transforming your menopausal symptoms.

4

TRANSFORMING YOUR
MENOPAUSE SYMPTOMS

Josie, a 53-year-old nurse, faced a tough menopause journey. Hot flashes made her feel insecure during work meetings, leaving her embarrassed and sweaty. But it wasn't just about the hot flashes.

Josie dealt with extreme anxiety. She worried a lot, withdrew from social interactions, and felt like everything was falling apart. Her once-strong confidence weakened, both at her job and in her role as a busy mom.

Josie saw her doctor, who diagnosed her with depression and prescribed antidepressants. But Josie suspected her mood swings were connected to her hormones. Josie wanted hormone replacement therapy (HRT), but concerns about breast cancer risk stopped her.

Despite some doctors advising against it, Josie persisted. She knew her risk wasn't as high as feared. In the end, HRT brought her relief. It changed her life, bringing back her happiness and self-assurance.

In this chapter, we'll dive into the fourth part of the 7 **RESTORE Steps to Gut Health**, which is all about Transforming your menopause symptoms.

Think about waking up in the morning feeling clear-headed, emotionally steady, and energized—despite the whirlwind of changes menopause brings. It might sound too good to be true, but the secret lies in an unexpected place: your gut. Yes, that complex system tasked with digesting your food holds incredible power over not just your physical health but also your mental and emotional well-being. By harnessing the gut-brain connection, you can navigate menopause more smoothly and feel your best every day.

In this chapter, we'll uncover how a healthy gut can ease your menopause symptoms and bring about improvements in your mental and emotional health. You'll learn about the complex gut-brain connection and why it's essential for your overall well-being. We will also investigate practical strategies to support gut health. This chapter will equip you with the knowledge you need to change your menopause journey into a period of empowered, vibrant living.

TACKLING YOUR MENOPAUSE SYMPTOMS WITH A HEALTHY GUT

Menopause can feel like your body is going rogue, throwing all sorts of curveballs your way. The hot flashes, mood swings, and anxiety are bad enough, but then your gut decides to join the rebellion too. Suddenly, you're bloated, constipated, and feeling like your once-faithful stomach has committed mutiny.

The culprit? Those ever-changing hormone levels during menopause don't just mess with your reproductive system; they wreak havoc on your gut health too. An inflamed or out-of-balance gut microbiome can send distress signals straight to your brain, making you feel more stressed, down in the dumps, and more emotionally up and down than a seesaw at a playground.

It's a vicious cycle—the hormonal chaos fuels gut issues, which then exacerbate the emotional roller coaster you're already riding. Pretty soon, this natural phase of life can start to feel overwhelming, unmanageable, and like your body has declared war on you from the inside out. But don't surrender just yet! Understanding this brain-gut connection is key to finding ways to restore balance during menopause.

UNDERSTANDING THE GUT-BRAIN CONNECTION

The gut-brain connection is one of the most fascinating and complex relationships within our bodies. It's a two-way street, a constant conversation happening between your gut and your brain. This partnership impacts everything from your digestion to your emotional well-being.

They're continually exchanging messages through a complex system scientists call the gut-brain axis. It's a superhighway that runs both ways, with information zipping back and forth at lightning speed.

At its core, the brain-gut connection involves a network of neurons, chemicals, and hormones that continually send signals back and forth between your gut and your brain. The enteric nervous system (ENS), often called "the second brain," is a critical player here. Believe it or not, you've got millions of nerve cells lining your digestive tract from your esophagus down to your rectum. This ENS controls the mechanics of digestion, but it's also a huge influencer on your mood and mindset.

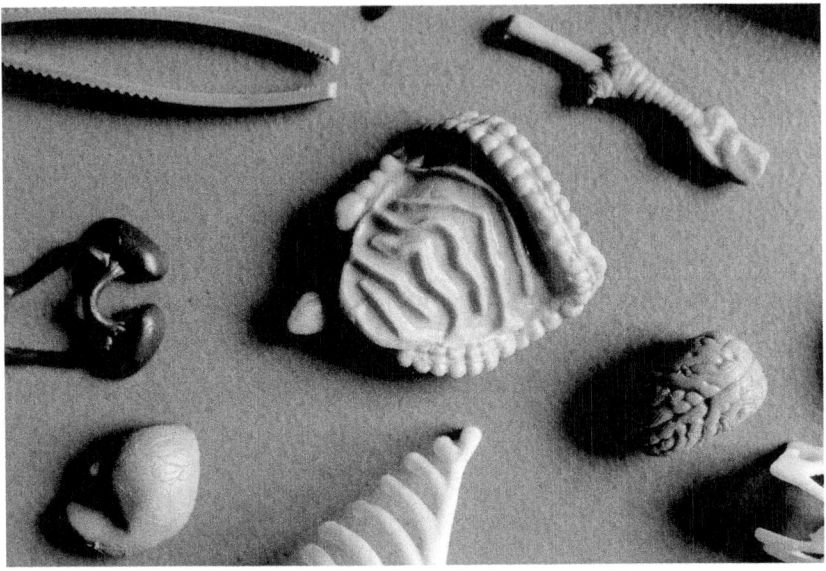

Then you've got the vagus nerve, which acts like a walkie-talkie connecting your gut straight to your brain stem. This nerve regulates involuntary functions like heart rate and digestion while also playing air traffic controller for your body's stress responses and emotional regulation.

But wait, there's more! The trillions of microbes living in your intestines that make up your gut microbiome are key communicators too. These tiny guys produce neurotransmitters like serotonin and dopamine—you know, the feel-good chemicals that help stabilize your mood and mental health. When this microbiome is out of balance, it can seriously throw off your emotional equilibrium.

Why the Gut-Brain Connection Is Important for Gut Health

Why is the teamwork between the brain and the gut so important? Beyond just keeping your digestion running smoothly, this connection ensures your brain is looped in on your body's nutritional needs. It's like having a direct line to the drive-thru worker so your order (nutrients) never gets messed up.

This partnership is important during menopause when those hormonal shifts can make you feel like your brain and gut are staging an all-out civil war. An inflamed gut will dispatch distress signals to your brain, which can amp up anxiety, depression, mood swings—all the fun stuff.

From your ENS choreographing digestion to your vagus nerve moderating stress responses based on gut cues, this gut-brain collaboration impacts everything from your appetite to emotional volatility. And when this connection goes haywire during menopause, it can seriously disrupt your physical and mental well-being.

THE GUT-BRAIN CONNECTION AND MENTAL CONDITIONS

Which mental conditions are tied to the gut-brain connection? Mainly we're looking at anxiety and depression, but the link extends to other conditions like IBS and even Alzheimer's disease. When your gut is unhealthy, it can worsen these issues.

Supporting a healthy gut is a powerful strategy for improving mental and emotional well-being, particularly during menopause. Here are some ways to achieve this:

- **Focus on maintaining a balanced diet:** A diet rich in fiber, lean proteins, and fermented foods like yogurt and kefir promotes good bacteria in your gut.
- **Consider taking probiotics or prebiotics:** Probiotics introduce beneficial bacteria into your digestive system, and prebiotics feed the existing good bacteria.
- **Manage stress:** Activities like yoga, meditation, or simple breathing exercises can help you manage your stress. Stress can severely impact your gut health and by extension your mental well-being.
- **Stay hydrated:** Water aids with digestion and helps maintain the mucosal lining of the intestines, which is crucial for a healthy gut.
- **Get adequate sleep:** Quality sleep is integral to both gut health and mental clarity.

When your gut is functioning well, you're better equipped to handle physical and emotional challenges along with menopause. Balanced gut bacteria can reduce systemic inflammation, which in turn eases anxiety and depression symptoms. Moreover, improved gut health often translates to better nutrient absorption, providing your brain with the essential vitamins and minerals it needs to function optimally.

Your gut deserves attention, care, and respect just as much as any other part of your body. Let's listen to what our guts are telling us, shall we?

HOW A HEALTHY GUT SUPPORTS A HEALTHY MIND

Nurturing a healthy brain-gut connection also depends on the foods and supplements you choose. Let's explore some key players in this dynamic relationship to understand why they are beneficial.

- **Probiotics:** Often associated with yogurt and other fermented foods, probiotics are live microorganisms that provide numerous health benefits, as we discussed in Chapter 3. They help maintain a balanced gut flora, which is essential for optimal digestive health. Research also indicates that a balanced gut can positively impact your mood and cognitive function by producing neurotransmitters like serotonin, often called the "happy hormone."

- **Omega-3 fats and other healthy fats:** Omega-3 fatty acids found in fish such as salmon and mackerel, chia seeds, and flaxseeds have been shown to support cognitive health and reduce inflammation. These fats are essential as they form part of brain cell membranes and have anti-inflammatory properties, which help in reducing gut inflammation, thus supporting a strong brain-gut link.

- **Fermented foods:** We learned in Chapter 3 that foods like sauerkraut, kimchi, kefir, and kombucha are rich in probiotics and can enhance gut health significantly. Fermented foods not only introduce beneficial bacteria into the gut but also create an acidic environment where harmful bacteria cannot thrive. This promotes a more stable gut environment conducive to good brain health.

- **High-fiber foods:** We have already mentioned that fiber is crucial for maintaining gut health. It acts as a prebiotic by feeding the good bacteria in your gut. High-fiber foods include fruits, vegetables, legumes, and whole grains. A fiber-rich diet has been associated with lower rates of depression and anxiety, indicating a positive brain-gut interaction.

- **Polyphenol-rich foods:** Polyphenols are antioxidants found in foods like berries, dark chocolate, olive oil, and green tea. They support gut and brain health by reducing inflammation and oxidative stress. Incorporating polyphenol-rich foods can protect against neurodegenerative diseases and improve mental well-being.

- **Tryptophan-rich foods:** Tryptophan is an amino acid essential for the production of serotonin. Foods high in tryptophan, such as turkey, eggs, tofu, and nuts, can boost serotonin levels in the brain, thus enhancing mood and emotional stability.
- **Mushrooms:** Certain types of mushrooms, such as reishi, shiitake, and maitake, contain prebiotics that nurture beneficial gut bacteria. They also offer immune-supporting properties that contribute to overall gut integrity, indirectly supporting brain health.
- **Nuts:** Almonds, walnuts, and cashews are packed with essential nutrients, including omega-3 fatty acids, antioxidants, and fiber. Regular consumption can bolster gut health and support cognitive function.
- **Sesame seeds:** These tiny seeds are nutritional powerhouses loaded with fiber, healthy fats, and magnesium. They can aid in regulating gut motility and improving gut flora, fostering a robust brain-gut connection.

Important Mindful Eating Tips

You can incorporate these foods into your diet along with these other dietary recommendations:

- Start your day with a breakfast smoothie made from yogurt for probiotics, chia seeds for omega-3s, and berries for polyphenols.

- Add a variety of vegetables to your lunch and dinner to ensure you get plenty of fiber.
- Snack on a handful of nuts or a piece of dark chocolate during the day.
- Include fish or a plant-based omega-3 source, like flaxseeds or algae oil, a few times a week.
- Experiment with fermented foods; a side of sauerkraut or kimchi can brighten up any meal.

Supporting a healthy brain-gut connection goes beyond diet. Here are some tips to guide you in achieving this goal:

- **Eat a variety of foods:** Diversity in your diet ensures you're getting a wide range of nutrients necessary for both gut and brain health. Various foods feed different kinds of beneficial gut bacteria, promoting a balanced microbiome.
- **Avoid gluten and processed foods:** Some people find that gluten and highly processed foods exacerbate gut issues, which can negatively affect mental health. Opting for whole, minimally processed foods can make a significant difference.
- **Work on improving your mental health and your gut health:** Practices such as mindfulness, meditation, and regular physical activity can help lower stress and anxiety, which in turn supports better gut health.
- **Reconnect and experience a sense of safety:** Engaging in activities and relationships that make you feel safe and connected can have a profound effect on both mental health and gut function. Consider spending time with loved ones, practicing yoga, or walking in nature.

- **Rule out infections:** Sometimes persistent gut issues can be due to underlying infections. Consulting a healthcare provider to rule out or treat infections is crucial for maintaining a healthy gut-brain axis.
- **Stay hopeful:** Maintaining a positive outlook can be powerful. Positive emotions and attitudes can directly influence gut health, creating a beneficial cycle of well-being.

Through mindful eating and integrating these practices into your life, you can support a healthy brain-gut connection and alleviate various menopause symptoms. It's all about balance—taking little steps toward a healthier lifestyle can cumulatively have a big impact. Embrace the journey toward well-being with optimism and kindness toward yourself.

THE MENOPAUSE WAY OF LIFE

The menopause diet is designed specifically to help manage symptoms associated with this natural stage of life. At its core, it's about eating foods that support hormonal balance, bone health, and overall well-being while avoiding those that can exacerbate symptoms. Understanding what to eat and what to avoid can make a significant difference in how you feel daily.

What to Include in Your Plan

Creating a well-balanced nutrition plan during menopause is necessary for managing your symptoms and maintaining overall health. Your plan should focus on key nutrients and food groups that address the specific challenges of this life stage. In the following sections, we'll explore the critical components to include.

Calcium-Rich Foods

During menopause, calcium becomes crucial. As estrogen levels drop, bones can lose density, increasing the risk of osteoporosis. Dairy products like milk, cheese, and yogurt are excellent sources of calcium. If you're lactose intolerant or prefer nondairy options, fortified plant-based milk and leafy greens such as kale and broccoli also provide substantial amounts of calcium.

Vegetables and Fruits

Rich in essential vitamins, minerals, and antioxidants, vegetables and fruits should be at the heart of your menopause diet. They contribute to overall health, improve digestion, and can help manage weight. Aim for a colorful plate—think berries, citrus fruits, bell peppers, and dark leafy greens—as each color offers different beneficial compounds.

Lean Protein

Including lean protein in your meals helps maintain muscle mass, which can decline with age and hormonal changes. Opt for chicken, turkey, fish, eggs, beans, and legumes. These sources of protein are not only important for muscle upkeep but also help keep you feeling full longer, reducing unnecessary snacking.

Soy Products

Soy contains phytoestrogens—plant-based compounds that mimic estrogen in the body. Incorporating soy products like tofu, tempeh, and edamame can help balance hormone levels naturally, potentially easing hot flashes and night sweats.

Iron-Rich Foods

Iron is vital for maintaining energy levels and preventing anemia, especially if menstrual periods are still occurring sporadically during perimenopause. Include iron-rich foods such as red meat, poultry, lentils, spinach, and fortified cereals in your diet.

Fiber-Rich Foods

Again, a fiber-rich diet supports digestive health, which can be particularly important during menopause, when digestion may slow down. Whole grains, fruits, vegetables, nuts, seeds, and legumes are all excellent sources of fiber. Not only does fiber aid in regular bowel movements, but it also helps control blood sugar levels and may reduce cholesterol.

Vitamin D Supplements

While some foods contain Vitamin D, it's often challenging to get enough from diet alone. Vitamin D helps with calcium absorption and bone health. Spending time outdoors in sunlight can boost vitamin D levels, but a supplement is often necessary, especially in less sunny climates or during winter months.

Healthy Fats

Healthy fats, such as those found in avocados, nuts, seeds, and fatty fish like salmon, are crucial for brain health, hormone production, and reducing inflammation. They can also help maintain satiety and prevent overeating.

Whole Grains

Whole grains should be included in your diet for their fiber content and ability to stabilize blood sugar levels. Options like quinoa, brown rice, oats, and whole wheat products can provide sustained energy without causing spikes in blood sugar.

Phytoestrogen-Containing Foods

Besides soy, other foods like flaxseeds, sesame seeds, and certain legumes also contain phytoestrogens. These can have a mild regulatory effect on your hormones. Including them regularly in your diet might help alleviate some of the more uncomfortable menopause symptoms.

What to Exclude From Your Plan

In contrast to the foods you need to consider incorporating into your lifestyle that we discussed in the last section, certain foods should be avoided to minimize menopause symptoms.

Spicy Foods

Spicy foods can trigger hot flashes and night sweats in many women. It might be helpful to limit or eliminate foods spiced with chili peppers, hot sauces, and other fiery ingredients.

Caffeine and Alcohol

Both caffeine and alcohol can interfere with sleep and worsen hot flashes. Reducing intake or cutting these out entirely might make a noticeable difference in your comfort levels. Try substituting herbal teas and mocktails as alternatives.

Carbs and Starchy Foods

Simple carbohydrates and starchy foods can cause rapid spikes and drops in blood sugar levels, leading to mood swings and energy crashes. Cut back on white bread, pasta, pastries, and sugary snacks. Opt instead for complex carbs, such as those found in whole grains.

Sugary and Salty Foods

Foods high in sugar and salt can contribute to bloating, weight gain, and water retention. Read labels and try to choose fresh, whole foods over processed ones. Be mindful of hidden sugars and salts in packaged foods and seasonings.

High-Fat Foods

Highly processed, high-fat foods are generally low in nutrients and can lead to weight gain, which exacerbates menopause symptoms. Focus on healthy fats from natural sources rather than fried or heavily processed foods.

Staying Hydrated Matters

Staying hydrated is equally important during menopause. Water aids in digestion, keeps skin hydrated, and helps regulate body temperature. Make it a habit to drink plenty of water throughout the day. You might find carrying a reusable water bottle with you helps you track your intake. Herbal teas and fresh juices with no added sugar also count toward your hydration goals.

Incorporating this diet with tips from the previous chapter can yield even better results. Here are some ways to do it:

- Integrate small portions of the recommended foods into each meal.
- Plan your weekly menu around the key components of the menopause diet to ensure variety and balance.
- Prepare snacks ahead of time that fit within these guidelines to avoid reaching for unhealthy options.

- Remain flexible and listen to your body, adjusting your diet as needed to best suit your personal health needs and preferences.

GUT-BRAIN RECIPES TO HELP REDUCE MENOPAUSE SYMPTOMS

In Chapter 3 we have tried 25 recipes to boost our gut health. Now let's dive right into some more gut-friendly recipes that are packed with nutrients for your gut-brain environment and are menopause symptom-friendly!

Breakfast Recipes

Start your day with tasty combinations that help support your digestive health.

Recipe 26: Blueberry Chia Pudding

Ingredients & tools

- 3 tbsp chia seeds
- 1 cup unsweetened almond milk
- 1 tsp vanilla extract
- 1 tbsp maple syrup
- 1/2 cup fresh blueberries (or berries of choice)
- 1 tbsp collagen peptides
- Mason jar or bowl and whisk

Instructions

- Combine the chia seeds, almond milk, vanilla extract, and maple syrup in mason jar or bowl.
- Whisk everything together until blended well.
- Let it sit for about 10 minutes, then give it another whisk to break up any clumps.
- Cover and refrigerate overnight or at least 4 hours.
- Serve with fresh berries on top.

Why this is good for menopause symptoms

Chia seeds are packed with omega-3 fatty acids known to reduce inflammation. The fiber helps support gut health, which is vital as menopause can cause digestive issues. Blueberries offer antioxidants that improve cognitive function, potentially mitigating mood swings.

Collagen helps improve skin elasticity and reduce wrinkles, addressing one of the common cosmetic concerns during menopause due to declining estrogen levels. It also supports joint health and reduces joint pain, which can be exacerbated by hormonal changes during menopause.

<u>Recipe 27: Spinach and Mushroom Omelet</u>

Ingredients & tools

- 2 eggs
- Handful of spinach
- 3–4 mushrooms, sliced
- Salt and pepper to taste
- Olive oil spray
- Nonstick frying pan and spatula

Instructions

- Whisk the eggs in a bowl, adding salt and pepper.
- Spray the frying pan with olive oil and warm up over medium heat.
- Add the mushrooms and cook until they soften, then add spinach.
- Pour the eggs over the vegetables and cook until set, flipping halfway through.

Why this is good for menopause symptoms

Eggs provide high-quality protein and vitamin D, which support bone health. Spinach is rich in iron and magnesium, aiding in energy levels and reducing fatigue.

Recipe 28: Filled Avocado Salad

Ingredients & tools

- 2 tbsp orange or lemon juice
- 1 large avocado
- 1/4 cup strawberries
- 1/4 cup blueberries
- 1/4 cup blackberries
- 1/2 cup cooked or raw broccoli
- 1 tbsp nuts, chopped
- 2 tbsp balsamic vinaigrette
- Cutting board, bowl, knife, and spoon.

Instructions

- Rinse the fruit with clean water and pat dry on a paper towel.
- Wash the broccoli and chop it into bite-size pieces.
- Slice the avocado in half and remove its pit. Paint 1 tbsp of orange or lemon juice over it to prevent it from turning brown.
- Stir the remaining juice with 1 tbsp of balsamic vinaigrette. Mix the fruit and broccoli together with the juice and balsamic mixture. Next, fill the avocado halves.
- Drizzle the rest of the balsamic reduction on top before serving.

Why this is good for menopause symptoms

Avocados are rich in healthy fats and fiber, promoting satiety and healthy digestion. Broccoli, nuts, and berries are good for your brain and body too.

Recipe 29: Plain Yogurt with Nuts and Honey

Ingredients & tools

- 1 cup plain yogurt (preferably Greek)
- Handful of mixed nuts
- 1 tbsp honey
- Measuring cups and spoon

Instructions

- Put the plain yogurt into a bowl.
- Sprinkle mixed nuts over the yogurt.

- Drizzle honey on top

Why this is good for menopause symptoms

Plain yogurt (like Greek yogurt) offers probiotics that are beneficial for gut health. The combination of protein and healthy fats from the nuts helps stabilize blood sugar levels, while honey adds a natural sweetness without causing a sugar spike.

Recipe 30: Quinoa Breakfast Bowl

Ingredients & tools

- 1/2 cup cooked quinoa
- 1 banana, sliced
- 1 tbsp almond butter
- 1 tsp chia seeds
- Small saucepan and bowl

Instructions

- Cook the quinoa according to package instructions if not precooked.
- Place the warm quinoa in a bowl and top with banana slices, almond butter, and chia seeds.

Why this is good for menopause symptoms

Quinoa is a complete protein and high in fiber, supporting digestive health. Bananas provide potassium to control blood pressure, and almond butter adds healthy fats essential for hormonal balance.

Lunch Recipes

Keep your energy up with these fresh and delicious lunch recipes!

Recipe 31: Grilled Chicken Salad

Ingredients & tools

- 1 chicken breast
- 1 cup mixed greens
- 1 tomato, chopped
- 1/2 cucumber, sliced
- 1/4 red onion, thinly sliced
- Olive oil, balsamic vinegar, salt, and pepper
- Grill or stovetop pan and salad bowl

Instructions

- Season the chicken breast with salt and pepper.
- Grill or pan-sear chicken until fully cooked, then slice into strips.
- Mix the greens, tomato, cucumber, and red onion in a bowl.
- Top with grilled chicken and drizzle with olive oil and balsamic vinegar.

Why this is good for menopause symptoms

Lean protein from chicken helps maintain muscle mass, which is important as metabolism slows down during menopause. Fresh vegetables supply essential vitamins and minerals that combat fatigue and support mental clarity.

Recipe 32: Lentil Soup

Ingredients & tools

- 1 cup lentils, rinsed
- 1 carrot, diced
- 1 celery stalk, diced
- 1 onion, chopped
- 2 garlic cloves, minced
- 4 cups vegetable broth
- 1 tsp cumin
- Salt and pepper to taste
- Large pot and ladle

Instructions

- In a large pot, sauté onions, carrots, celery, and garlic until soft.
- Add lentils, broth, cumin, salt, and pepper.
- Bring to a boil, then simmer for 30 minutes or until lentils are tender.

Why this is good for menopause symptoms

Lentils are full of fiber and protein, aiding in digestive health and maintaining blood sugar stability. They also provide iron, which is crucial for fighting menopause-related fatigue.

Recipe 33: Tofu Stir-Fry

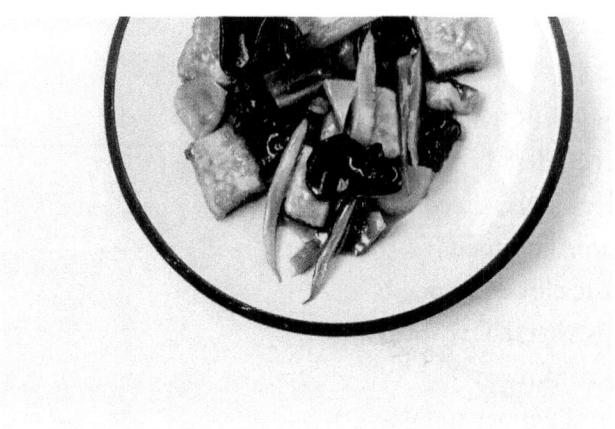

Ingredients & tools

- 1 block of firm tofu
- 1 bell pepper, sliced
- 1 broccoli head, cut into florets
- 1 carrot, julienned
- soy sauce
- olive oil
- 1 tsp garlic, chopped
- 1 tsp fresh or ground ginger
- Wok or large skillet and spatula

Instructions

- Cube the tofu.
- Heat oil in a wok, adding garlic and ginger.
- Stir-fry the tofu until golden brown, remove, and set aside.
- In the same wok, stir-fry vegetables until tender-crisp.
- Return tofu to the wok, add soy sauce, and mix well.

- You can be creative with the vegetables and use what is available to you. Make sure you opt for low-glycemic index (GI) veggies by doing an online search for their GI score.

Why this is good for menopause symptoms

Tofu provides plant-based protein and phytoestrogens, which can help balance hormones. The colorful veggies are rich in antioxidants that combat oxidative stress.

Recipe 34: Mediterranean Chickpea Salad

Ingredients & tools

- 1 can chickpeas, drained
- 1 cucumber, diced
- 1 tomato, diced
- 1/4 red onion, finely chopped
- 1/4 cup feta cheese, crumbled
- Olive oil, lemon juice, salt, and pepper
- Mixing bowl and spoon

Instructions

- Combine chickpeas, cucumber, tomato, onion, and feta in a mixing bowl.
- Drizzle with olive oil and lemon juice.
- Season with salt and pepper, mix well and serve.

Why this is good for menopause symptoms

Chickpeas are high in fiber and plant proteins, helping with digestive regularity and satiety. The Mediterranean diet's principles can alleviate various menopause symptoms with balanced nutrition.

Recipe 35: Salmon and Avocado Wrap

Ingredients & tools

- 1 whole wheat tortilla
- 1 salmon fillet, cooked and flaked
- 1/2 avocado, sliced
- 1 cup mixed greens
- Lemon juice, salt, and pepper
- Frying pan and spatula

Instructions

- Warm the tortilla in a pan.
- Lay out the mixed greens on the tortilla and place the salmon and avocado slices on top.
- Drizzle with lemon juice and sprinkle with salt and pepper.
- Roll the tortilla and serve.

Why this is good for menopause symptoms

Salmon is an excellent source of omega-3 fatty acids, which support brain health and reduce inflammation. Avocado provides healthy fats that are good for hormone production.

Dinner Recipes

These dinner recipes will help keep you full and your gut happy.

Recipe 36: Baked Cod with Asparagus

Ingredients & tools

- 2 cod fillets
- 1 bunch asparagus, trimmed
- Olive oil, lemon zest, salt, and pepper
- Baking sheet, parchment paper, and oven

Instructions

- Preheat oven to 375 °F (190 °C).
- Place cod and asparagus on a baking sheet lined with parchment paper.
- Drizzle with olive oil and sprinkle with lemon zest, salt, and pepper.
- Bake for 15–20 minutes or until cod is flaky.

Why this is good for menopause symptoms

Cod is low-calorie and high-protein, aiding muscle maintenance. Asparagus is a good source of fiber and contains folate, which supports mood regulation.

<u>Recipe 37: Quinoa-Stuffed Bell Peppers</u>

Ingredients & tools

- 4 bell peppers
- 1 cup cooked quinoa
- 1/2 cup black beans, rinsed
- 1 tomato, chopped
- 1/2 cup corn kernels
- Cumin, chili powder, salt, and pepper
- Baking dish and foil

Instructions

- Preheat oven to 375 °F (190 °C).
- Slice tops off bell peppers and remove seeds.
- Mix quinoa, black beans, tomato, corn, and spices in a bowl.
- Stuff each bell pepper with the mixture and place in a baking dish.
- Cover with foil and bake for 30 minutes.

Why this is good for menopause symptoms

These stuffed peppers are fiber-rich and loaded with plant proteins, maintaining stable blood glucose levels. They're also easy on the digestive system.

Recipe 38: Garlic Shrimp with Zoodles

Ingredients & tools

- 1 lb shrimp, peeled and deveined
- 3 zucchinis, spiralized
- 3 garlic cloves, minced
- Olive oil, parsley, salt, and pepper
- Spiralizer, frying pan, and tongs

Instructions

- Using the spiralizer, turn the zucchini into noodles (zoodles). Set aside.
- Heat olive oil in a pan and sauté garlic until fragrant.
- Add shrimp and cook until pink, about 3–4 minutes per side.
- Remove shrimp and set aside. Add zoodles to the pan and cook briefly.
- Return shrimp to the pan, toss with zoodles, and season with salt, pepper, and parsley.

Why this is good for menopause symptoms

Shrimp provides lean protein and zinc for immune health. Zoodles are a low-carb alternative to pasta, boosting veggie intake without the carbohydrate load.

Recipe 39: Turmeric Cauliflower Curry

Ingredients & tools

- 1 head cauliflower, broken into florets
- 1 can coconut milk
- 1 onion, chopped
- 3 garlic cloves, minced
- 1 tsp turmeric
- 1 tsp curry powder
- 1 tsp cumin
- Salt to taste
- Large pot and wooden spoon

Instructions

- Sauté onion and garlic until translucent.
- Add turmeric, curry powder, cumin, and salt. Cook for another minute.
- Stir in cauliflower and coconut milk and bring to a simmer.
- Cook for 15–20 minutes until cauliflower is tender.

Why this is good for menopause symptoms

Curcumin in turmeric is anti-inflammatory and may aid in reducing menopausal joint pain. This dish also promotes gut health with its fiber content.

Recipe 40: Chicken and Vegetable Skewers

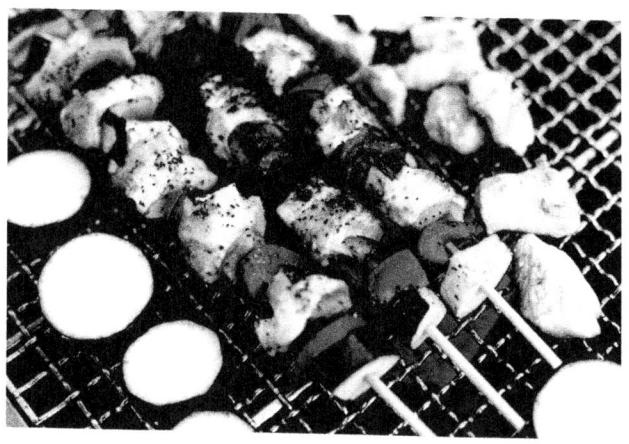

Ingredients & tools

- 2 chicken breasts, cubed
- 24 cherry tomatoes (about 2 cups)
- 2 medium bell peppers, cut into 1-in. squares
- 1 large zucchini, cut into 1/2-in.-thick rounds
- Olive oil, salt, pepper, and oregano to taste
- Skewers and grill or broiler

Instructions

- Thread chicken and veggies onto skewers.
- Drizzle with olive oil and sprinkle with salt, pepper, and oregano.
- Grill or broil for about 15 minutes, turning occasionally, until chicken is cooked.

Why this is good for menopause symptoms

Balanced with lean protein and a variety of veggies, this meal offers comprehensive nutrition. It supports muscle health and provides necessary vitamins and minerals.

Dessert & Snack Recipes

These quick sweet treats will keep you going between meals without disrupting your gut.

Recipe 41: Dark Chocolate Almond Bark

Ingredients & tools

- 1 cup dark chocolate chips
- 1/2 cup almonds, chopped
- Microwave-safe bowl and baking sheet

Instructions

- Melt chocolate chips in the microwave using a microwave-safe bowl.
- Stir in chopped almonds.
- Spread mixture on a baking sheet and refrigerate until set.
- Break into pieces and enjoy.

Why this is good for menopause symptoms

This is a satisfying and nutritious snack that can help manage cravings and mood swings. Dark chocolate contains antioxidants that may help reduce inflammation. Almonds are a good source of vitamin E, which can help alleviate hot flashes and other menopausal symptoms.

Recipe 42: Almond Protein Fig Bars

Ingredients & tools

- 1 tbsp flax meal
- 2 tbsp raw honey
- 1 cup almond butter
- 2 scoops of vanilla-flavored bone broth protein powder or vanilla-flavored collagen peptides
- 1 cup dried figs

Instructions

- Begin by lining an 8x8 baking sheet with parchment paper.
- Combine all the ingredients in a food processor and blend until a dough forms.
- Press the dough evenly into the prepared pan and refrigerate for at least 2 hours until set.
- Once set, cut into squares and store in an airtight container. Makes 12 servings.

Why this is good for menopause symptoms

This recipe is good for gut-brain health because figs are high in fiber, almond butter provides healthy fats, flax meal is rich in omega-3 fatty acids, collagen peptides support gut health, and raw honey contains beneficial antioxidants, which are also good for managing menopause symptoms.

Recipe 43: Lemon Tart

Ingredients & tools

Crust:

- 1/2 tsp sea salt
- 2 tbsp melted coconut oil
- 2 cups blanched almond flour
- 1–2 eggs

Lemon curd:

- 2 tbsp lemon zest
- 1/2 cup fresh lemon juice
- 4 eggs at room temperature
- 2 scoops collagen protein
- 1/2 cup maple syrup
- 1/2 tsp sea salt
- 1/2 cup coconut oil or unsalted butter
- Mixed berries and thinly sliced lemons (optional toppings)

Instructions

- Preheat the oven to 350 °F (180 °C) and lightly grease a 9-in. tart pan.
- Combine almond flour, sea salt, melted coconut oil, and egg in a food processor or mixing bowl until a ball forms.
- Press the dough into the tart pan, prick it with a fork, place parchment paper and a pie weight on top, then bake for 10–15 minutes until golden. Let it cool for 15 minutes.
- In a saucepan, whisk together lemon zest, lemon juice, eggs, maple syrup, collagen protein, and salt.

- Add coconut oil or butter over low heat, whisking constantly for about 5 minutes, then increase heat and whisk for 15–20 minutes until the curd thickens.
- Remove from heat and cool for 10 minutes.
- Transfer the lemon curd to a glass container, cover, and refrigerate for at least 2 hours or overnight.
- Pour the lemon curd over the cooled crust and bake for 15 minutes until set but jiggly in the center.
- Let it cool to room temperature, then chill in the refrigerator for at least 3 hours or overnight.
- Top with sliced lemons and mixed berries if desired.
- Slice, serve, and refrigerate any leftovers for up to a week or freeze to enjoy later.

Why this is good for menopause symptoms

Almond flour and coconut oil are easier to digest compared to traditional wheat flour and can help maintain gut health.

The lemon and collagen protein offer antioxidants and collagen support, which can be beneficial for skin elasticity and joint health during menopause.

Recipe 44: Oatmeal Cookies

Ingredients & tools

- 1 cup oats
- 1 banana, mashed
- 1/4 cup raisins
- Baking sheet and oven

Instructions

- Preheat oven to 350 °F (180 °C).
- Mix oats, mashed banana, and raisins in a bowl.
- Drop spoonfuls onto a baking sheet and bake for 15 minutes.

Why this is good for menopause symptoms

Oats are great for digestion, and bananas add natural sweetness and potassium, helpful for managing blood pressure.

Recipe 45: Hummus and Veggies

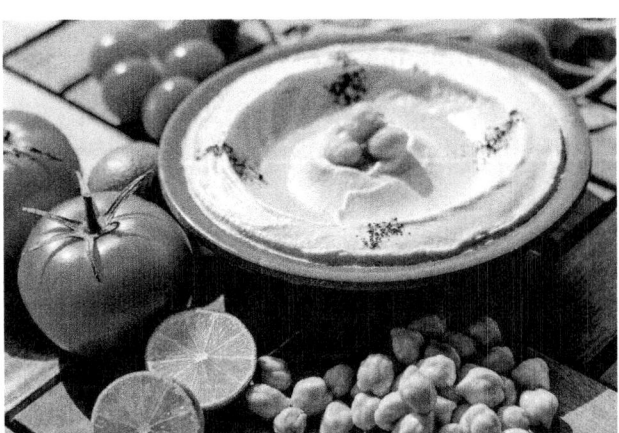

Ingredients & tools

- 1 cup hummus
- 2 medium carrots, cut into sticks
- 1 medium bell pepper, sliced
- 1/2 medium cucumber, cut into spears
- 6–8 cherry tomatoes
- Knife and plate

Instructions

- Slice veggies into sticks.
- Serve with hummus for dipping.

Why this is good for menopause symptoms

Made from chickpeas, hummus offers protein and fiber. Paired with veggies, it makes for a satisfying and nutrient-dense snack that aids in digestion and overall wellness.

Adding these recipes to your daily routine can enhance your gut health and alleviate menopause symptoms. We've learned that balancing nutrient-dense foods with good fats and fiber is key to managing and improving your well-being during this phase.

From the above recipes, you have learned why different foods are good for your gut health and menopause symptoms. With this knowledge, you can also mix and twist to create your own gut health recipes to enjoy!

In the next chapter, we will focus on optimizing your immunity and longevity with good digestive health.

5

OPTIMIZING YOUR IMMUNITY
AND LONGEVITY

As we go through menopause, we encounter hormonal shifts that can create a ripple effect throughout our entire body. One of the most impactful of these is the effect on our immune system.

Emily, a committed triathlete, was surprised by the changes in her body during perimenopause. She had always been active and loved her intense training sessions, but she experienced a sudden drop in energy levels, felt tired, had sore muscles, and lacked motivation.

Her immune system, which used to be strong, now seemed weaker. She found herself catching colds more frequently, taking longer to recover from minor illnesses, and even developing infections she'd never had before. What used to be a quick 24-hour bug now seemed to linger for days or even weeks.

Despite these challenges, Emily did not give up. She consulted healthcare professionals knowledgeable about perimenopause who explained how hormonal fluctuations affect the immune system. They highlighted the role of estrogen in influencing immune responses. As her estrogen levels decreased, her immune system's strength decreased as well.

With this new understanding, Emily made changes to her lifestyle. She focused on getting enough sleep, improving her diet, and reducing stress. She also added probiotics and prebiotics to support her gut health, indirectly benefiting her immune system.

Although it wasn't easy, Emily emerged from this journey stronger. Her immune system improved, allowing her to continue her athletic pursuits. Emily's experience teaches us that by understanding our bodies during menopause, we can make better choices for our health and well-being.

In this chapter, we'll explore the fifth step of the 7 **RESTORE Steps to Gut Health** focusing on **O**ptimizing your immunity and longevity by understanding the important link between gut health and immune function during menopause.

For many women, menopause brings about changes that are both physical and emotional, transforming day-to-day life in unexpected ways. An often overlooked aspect of this transition is the relationship between digestive health and overall well-being. Believe it or not, your gut plays a role in maintaining a strong immune system and promoting longevity, making it crucial to pay close attention to what happens internally during these pivotal years.

Reduced estrogen levels can weaken your immune response, making it easier for infections and illnesses to take hold. Think of your immune system as an army—its strength and readiness are partly influenced by hormones. When those fluctuate, it's like the army losing some of its key leaders, thereby becoming less effective. This weakened defense can lead to more frequent colds, longer recovery times, and increased susceptibility to chronic conditions like osteoporosis and heart disease.

Join me as I share some practical tips on nurturing gut health to boost your immune system.

IMMUNITY DURING MENOPAUSE

This may sound like something you win in a challenge on an episode of *Survivor*, but it's not. The only way to win immunity in the game of life—where we have absolutely no guarantees—is by making mindful choices that strengthen our immune systems.

You know, every day we make tons of choices about what to eat and drink. It can get pretty confusing with all the mixed messages out there about what's good for you and what's not. It's important to figure out what actually helps your body, not just what people claim is healthy.

The great news is that consuming the right nutrients can make a huge difference in your health—it might even extend your life! I get it, changing how you eat isn't always easy. But here's the thing: Lots of people have done it, and they found out it wasn't as hard as they thought. This is where you need to develop your resilience. Many even said that these healthier food choices tasted better than they ever expected!

As you start improving your nutrition, your taste buds actually wake up. Foods you maybe didn't like before might start tasting pretty good. It takes a while to get used to new foods, sure, but it's totally worth it in the long run. When you try out the tasty recipes shared in Chapters 3 and 4, you might find yourself actually loving this new way of eating!

What Role Does the Immune System Fulfill?

The immune system is your body's natural defense mechanism against infections and diseases. It is comprised of various cells, tissues, and organs that work harmoniously to identify and neutralize harmful pathogens like bacteria, viruses, and toxins. Key players in this complex network include white blood cells, antibodies, and other specialized components that patrol the body to keep threats at bay.

During menopause, the immune system undergoes notable changes that are influenced by hormonal shifts. Estrogen, a hormone that significantly impacts immune function, decreases substantially during menopause. This decline can lead to an altered immune response, making you more susceptible to infections and illnesses, especially when you reach the postmenopausal stage. This happens because estrogen enhances immune surveillance and modulates immune responses, essentially acting as a regulatory agent within this system.

When estrogen levels drop, there is a corresponding decrease in the efficiency of the immune system. The reduction in estrogen can lead to lower production of certain cytokines—proteins that play a crucial role in cell signaling within the immune system. These proteins help mediate and regulate immunity, inflammation, and hematopoiesis (blood formation). Lower levels of cytokines can result in weakened immune responses, making the body less effective at warding off infections. Menopause can increase your susceptibility to chronic conditions such as cardiovascular disease and osteoporosis, which can further strain the immune system.

We can't talk about your immune system without touching on autoimmune disorders—conditions where the immune system mistakenly attacks the body's tissues. Menopause can exacerbate or alter the course of these disorders. For instance, many women with autoimmune diseases like rheumatoid arthritis or lupus experience fluctuations in their symptoms during menopause. Hormonal changes can either trigger flare-ups or, conversely, bring periods of remission.

Some autoimmune diseases are more prevalent in women and tend to worsen around menopause. This pattern suggests that sex hormones, particularly estrogen, play a significant role in the incidence and severity of autoimmune conditions. The drop in estrogen levels can alter the balance of immune regulation, potentially leading to increased autoimmunity. Thus, understanding these hormonal influences is fundamental in managing autoimmune disorders during and after menopause.

HOW MENOPAUSE AFFECTS YOUR IMMUNE SYSTEM

During menopause, your body goes through hormonal changes, and these changes can weaken your immune system. It's like your army is suddenly missing some of its soldiers, so it becomes easier for germs—the enemy—to sneak in and cause trouble. This can make you more prone to getting sick or having health issues.

Fostering good digestive health is a key aspect that supports immunity and longevity. The gut houses a significant portion of the immune system, often referred to as the gut-associated lymphoid tissue (GALT).

BOOSTING YOUR IMMUNITY DURING MENOPAUSE

When your hormones change, some women find their bodies have a harder time fighting off sickness and staying healthy. Knowing how to improve your immune system during this time is important for going through menopause with energy and strength.

Exercise, Stress Management, and Sleep

Living a healthy lifestyle is crucial for maintaining a strong immune system during menopause. Regular exercise is like training for your immune army, keeping it strong and prepared for any battles that may come its way. Managing stress is also important to prevent your immune system from feeling overwhelmed. Think of sleep as giving your immune army a chance to regroup and recharge. By getting enough rest, you ensure your cellular soldiers are ready to face whatever challenges come their way the next day. We'll discuss this topic in more detail later in the chapter when we explore strategies for promoting longevity and mitigating the effects of aging.

Healthy Diet for Immunity

Eating a balanced diet rich in fruits, vegetables, and whole grains provides your immune system with the necessary nutrients and energy to ward off unwanted germs. These foods act as fuel for your immune soldiers, helping them stay strong in the fight against illnesses. Ensuring your body receives the right nourishment is like providing your army with the weapons and armor they need to protect your health.

Hydration for Overall Health

Proper hydration is vital for the optimal functioning of all your body's systems, including your immune system. Just like a well-oiled machine operates more smoothly, drinking plenty of water helps maintain your overall health. Hydration supports your immune army in carrying out its defensive duties effectively, ensuring you are guarded against infections and diseases.

SUPPLEMENTS TO BOOST IMMUNITY

Supporting your immune system during menopause can involve the use of certain supplements. Here are some examples of immune-friendly supplements that have shown promise in scientific studies:

- **Vitamin D:** Often called the "sunshine vitamin," vitamin D plays a crucial role in immune function. A meta-analysis by Martineau et al. found that vitamin D supplementation protected against acute respiratory tract infections (2017).
- **Vitamin C:** This antioxidant is well-known for its immune-boosting properties. A review published in 2017 by Carr and Maggini highlighted its role in supporting various cellular functions of the immune system.
- **Zinc:** This mineral is essential for the development and function of immune cells. A 2008 study by Prasad showed that zinc supplementation can help reduce the duration of common colds.
- **Elderberry:** Rich in antioxidants, elderberry has been shown to have antiviral properties. A study by Tiralongo et al. found that elderberry supplementation could reduce the severity and duration of cold and flu-like symptoms (2016).

- **Echinacea:** This herb has long been used to support immune health. A 2015 meta-analysis by Schapowal et al. suggested that echinacea could reduce the risk of recurrent respiratory infections.

Always consult with a healthcare provider before starting any new supplement regimen as individual needs can vary and some supplements may interact with medications or have side effects.

How a Healthy Gut Boosts Your Immunity

A healthy gut is important for general health, especially during menopause when your body's immune system can become more vulnerable. Research has shown that maintaining a healthy gut microbiome significantly boosts immunity, playing a pivotal role in defending the body against becoming unwell. We'll explore how a healthy gut microbiome supports a steady immune system both within and beyond the digestive tract in the following sections.

Immune System Regulation and Training

The gut microbiome educates and trains the immune system by exposing it to various antigens. This helps the immune system differentiate between harmful pathogens and harmless substances, reducing the risk of autoimmune diseases.

This microbiome regulates immune responses, ensuring that the body reacts appropriately to threats without causing excessive inflammation, which can lead to chronic diseases.

Barrier Function and Defense

A healthy gut lining acts as a barrier, preventing harmful pathogens and toxins from entering the bloodstream. The microbiome supports the integrity of this barrier, enhancing its protective function.

The gut microbiome stimulates GALT to produce immune cells like T-cells and B-cells, which are crucial for fighting infections.

Anti-Inflammatory Effects

Beneficial gut bacteria produce short-chain fatty acids (SCFAs) through the fermentation of dietary fibers. SCFAs have anti-inflammatory properties, which help modulate immune responses and reduce the risk of inflammatory diseases.

When you have a balanced microbiome, the production of pro-inflammatory cytokines—molecules that trigger or even increase inflammation   is kept in check, preventing chronic inflammation that can weaken the immune system.

Impact Beyond the Digestive Tract

The influence of a healthy gut microbiome extends beyond your digestive tract.

Respiratory Health

Research indicates a link between gut health and respiratory immunity. A balanced microbiome can enhance your immune response in the respiratory tract, providing better defense against respiratory infections, including the flu and common colds.

Systemic Immune Function

The gut microbiome interacts with various organs and systems through the bloodstream. Metabolites and signals from the gut can influence immune cells throughout the body, bolstering overall immune defense mechanisms.

Skin Health

The condition of the skin, the body's largest organ, is also linked to gut health. A healthy microbiome can reduce skin inflammation and improve conditions like eczema and psoriasis, indicating a systemic immune balance.

HOW GOOD DIGESTIVE HEALTH SUPPORTS LONGEVITY AND MITIGATES AGING

Researchers found that elderly persons who had a changing variety of intestinal bacterial composition throughout their lives tended to have increased longevity compared to those with more stable gut microbiomes (Wilmanski et al., 2021).

Good digestive health is necessary for living a longer, healthier life, especially during and after menopause. As women go through menopause, their bodies undergo numerous changes that can affect their overall health and how they age. Next, we'll explore how a healthy gut can be a cornerstone for aging gracefully and maintaining vitality.

Menopause and Its Impact on Aging and Longevity

The drop in estrogen levels that happens during menopause can influence various aspects of aging. This leads to

- decreased bone density, increasing the risk of osteoporosis and fractures.
- an increased risk of heart disease due to changes in cholesterol levels and blood vessel elasticity.
- a slower metabolism during menopause, which often leads to weight gain, especially around the abdomen, and can elevate the risk of chronic diseases.
- reduced estrogen, which can result in thinner, less elastic skin, leading to more pronounced wrinkles and sagging.

Menopause significantly impacts women's health and aging processes. Understanding these changes and supporting your digestive health can help you age more gracefully and stay healthier longer.

Want to learn more about navigating menopause and embracing anti-aging? Check out my book *The Ultimate Guide to Menopause Anti-Aging*. This comprehensive guide offers practical advice, expert insights, and strategies to help you feel your best during this life stage.

Tips to Adapt: Promoting Longevity and Mitigating Aging

Aging brings changes that can affect how we eat as well as what our bodies need, so we have to adapt in new ways. In this section, we'll explore some things you can do to add years to your life— one study even found that men who do these things by middle age can live up to 24 years longer and women up to 21 years longer (Lamontagne, 2023)!

Eat Like You Should

Your metabolism slows down with age, meaning your body needs fewer calories. Focus on nutrient-dense foods that provide the most bang for your buck in terms of vitamins and minerals. Eating a variety of plant-based foods like fruits, nuts, vegetables, seeds, whole grains, and beans can lower your risk of diseases and help you live longer.

Consuming a nutritious diet, especially one rich in plant-based foods, is linked to a lower risk of premature death and reduced risk of various diseases (Crichton-Stuart, 2023). Particularly advantageous for heart health is a Mediterranean-style diet, which is important since heart disease danger rises after menopause (Escobar, 2023).

- Taste and smell can diminish, making food less appealing. This may increase your inclination to add sugar or salt—a less healthy choice. Enhance flavors with herbs and spices instead.
- Eating smaller, more frequent meals can help if you have a reduced appetite. Include nutrient-dense snacks to maintain energy and nutrient levels.
- Stay hydrated, chew sugar-free gum, and eat moisture-rich foods like fruits and vegetables to combat dry mouth.
- If money is tight, plan meals, buy in bulk, and prioritize affordable, nutritious options like beans, lentils, and frozen vegetables.

Regular Eating Schedule

- Eating regular meals and snacks throughout the day can help prevent blood sugar fluctuations and maintain energy levels.
- Listen to your body's hunger and fullness cues to avoid overeating.

Food Safety Practices

- Follow safe food handling practices to prevent foodborne illnesses. Wash fruits and vegetables thoroughly, cook meat and poultry to the recommended temperatures, and refrigerate perishable foods promptly.
- Check expiration dates on food products to avoid consuming spoiled items.

Additional Tips

- If you're concerned about nutrient deficiencies, consult a healthcare professional about potential supplements.
- Stress can affect your digestion, which also affects your diet. Practice stress-reduction techniques like meditation, yoga, or deep breathing.
- Incorporate fiber-rich foods, such as fruits, vegetables, whole grains, and legumes, to promote regular bowel movements. Stay hydrated to prevent constipation.

Remember: While these tips can be helpful, it's essential to consult with a healthcare professional or registered dietitian for personalized advice based on your specific needs and health conditions.

Exercise Regularly

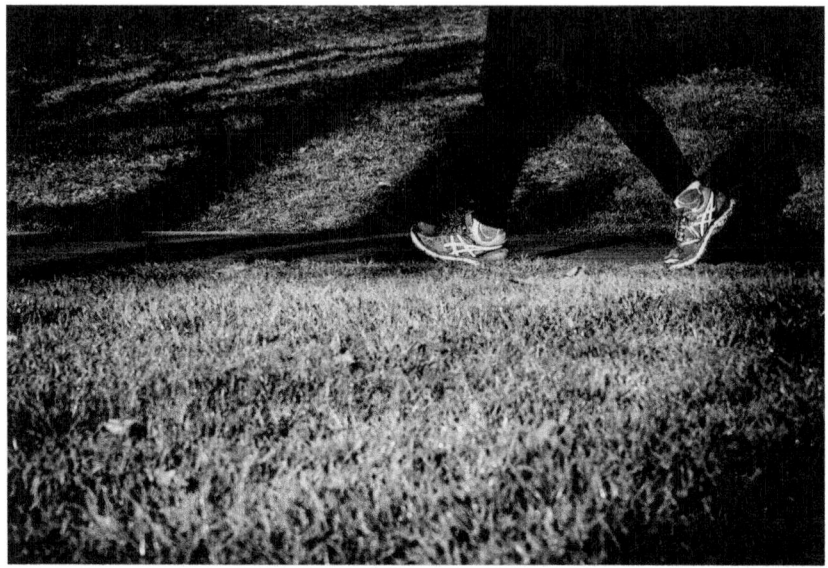

Exercise is a great way to reduce stress and improve your mood. Find an activity you enjoy, whether it's yoga, walking, dancing, or something else. Exercise releases endorphins, which are chemicals in your brain that make you feel good. Aim to incorporate physical activity into your routine a few times a week.

Engaging in exercise is associated with a longer, healthier life. Staying active can reduce the risk of developing illnesses, boost cognitive abilities, and promote a longer lifespan. Recent research that included more than 700,000 United States veterans revealed that individuals who incorporate eight healthy lifestyle habits by middle age can anticipate living significantly longer than those who practice few or none of these habits (Lamontagne, 2023). Engaging in physical activity can reduce the risk of developing long-term illnesses, boost cognitive performance, and promote a longer lifespan.

Stress Less

Stress can make you feel overwhelmed and tired. It is important to find ways to relax and stay positive. Managing stress and staying positive can help you live longer. Studies done in Japan showed that men who knew where they were going in life had fewer heart attacks and strokes than men who lacked self-confidence (Koizumi et al., 2008). Let's explore ways to improve your stress levels:

- **Positive thinking is key:** Having a good attitude toward life can help you in many ways. Try to remind yourself regularly of the good things in your life. This can help you feel better and reduce your stress levels. For example, if you feel sad, try to think of something that makes you happy, like a funny memory or a loved one.
- **Find your sense of direction:** Knowing what you want in life can make a big difference. Try to set goals for yourself, whether they are big or small. When you have goals, you have something to put your energy toward and look forward to. This can help you feel more positive about the future. For instance, if you want to learn a new skill, like cooking, you can set a goal to make a new recipe every week. This can give you a sense of accomplishment and purpose.
- **Take time for yourself:** It's essential to take time for yourself each day. This can help you relax and recharge. Find a hobby or activity you enjoy and make time for it regularly. It could be something simple like reading a book, going for a walk, or listening to music. Taking care of yourself is important for reducing stress and staying positive.

- **Practice mindfulness:** Mindfulness helps you be present in the moment. It involves paying attention to your thoughts and feelings without judging them. Mindfulness can help reduce stress and anxiety. Try to take a few minutes each day to sit quietly and focus on your breathing. This can help calm your mind and bring a sense of peace.

Stay Social

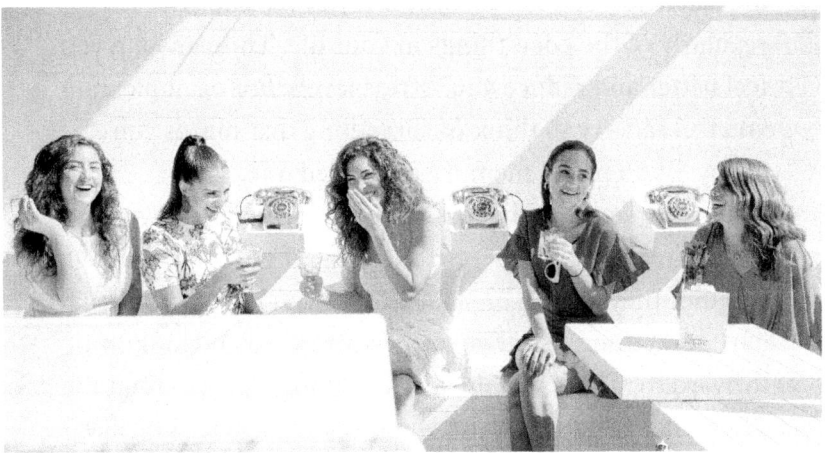

Talking to friends and family can also help reduce stress. Simply sharing your feelings with others can make you feel better. Reach out to someone you trust when you are feeling stressed or down. They might have advice or can just be there to listen. Having good friends and family around can boost your chances of living longer and staying healthy.

- Loneliness or depression can affect your eating habits. Try to eat with others, join social groups, and seek support to improve your mental well-being and nutrition.

- Having positive social relationships is associated with a longer lifespan. Maintaining healthy social networks can help promote longevity and decrease your risk of chronic diseases (Schimelpfening, 2023).

Get Enough Sleep

Sleep plays a vital role in various bodily functions, including cognitive performance, emotional well-being, and physical health. Getting eight hours of sleep every night can help increase your life (Petre, 2023).

Engage in Meaningful Hobbies and Activities

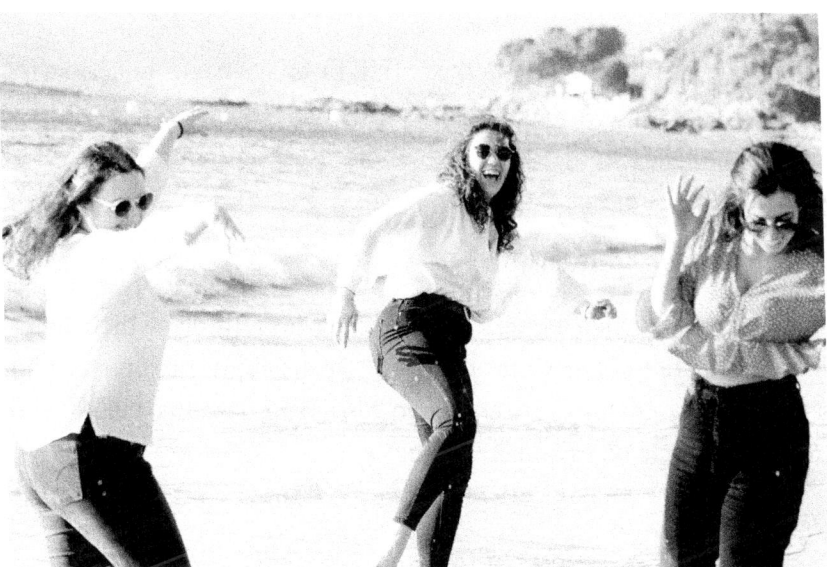

Spending time doing hobbies and activities that are meaningful to you can lengthen your life. Engaging in purposeful activities and self-reflection may help reduce the risk of Alzheimer's disease. Regularly asking yourself "why" you're doing certain activities encourages cognitive engagement, leading to more mindful behavior, which is associated with better brain health as you age.

Maintain a Healthy Weight

This is crucial for promoting longevity as obesity and being underweight can both have adverse effects on health. Slower digestion can lead to constipation, which may affect weight management. When your digestive system slows down, it can cause bloating, discomfort, and a temporary increase in your weight due to retained waste.

Increase your fiber intake, drink plenty of water, and stay active to keep things moving. Maintaining a balanced diet and engaging in regular physical activity are essential for achieving and sustaining a healthy weight.

Consider HRT

Hormone replacement therapy (HRT) may have benefits for longevity as it can relieve menopausal symptoms, reduce the risk of osteoporosis and certain other diseases, and improve overall well-being.

Improve Your Bone Health

Menopausal women benefit from strength training, which helps increase metabolic rate and maintain strong bones. Exercises that use body weight as resistance can also benefit bone health and increase muscle mass and strength.

Oral Hygiene

Menopause can be a bit of a troublemaker when it comes to the health of your teeth and gums. It might make you more likely to experience gum problems or even lose teeth. Yikes, right? But don't worry, it's not all doom and gloom. Stick to the basics—see your dentist regularly, brush those pearly whites, and don't forget to floss. It's like giving your mouth a little tender loving care every day.

Aging Skincare

Menopause can make your skin feel like it's gone through a desert —all dry and thin. But here's the good news: You can fight back! Use enough moisturizer (especially for dry skin), be gentle with your skin (no harsh chemicals!), and don't forget to protect it from the sun. Think of it like being your skin's best friend. With a little extra care, you can help your skin look and feel great.

Alcohol and Tobacco

Rethinking alcohol consumption and participating in tobacco cessation programs can have positive effects on health during menopause, such as reducing the risk of hot flashes and improving mental health challenges.

Manage Chronic Conditions Wisely

These conditions and associated medications to manage them can impact your appetite and digestion. Consult with your doctor to manage these effects and ensure you're meeting your nutritional needs.

Keep a Record of Your Cycle and Symptoms

Start a menstrual calendar and record your menopausal symptoms to help you notice patterns so you can better manage your symptoms.

Don't try to be perfect in any part of your life. It's impossible. Even when it comes to your gut, perfection isn't real. If you mess up in trying to improve your gut health, don't be too hard on yourself. Just get back up and try again.

AGING GRACEFULLY DURING MENOPAUSE

Menopause opens our eyes to the opportunity to age with strength and wisdom. Let's explore some tips for aging gracefully:

- **Stay informed:** When it comes to new information, be like a sponge. Talk to your doctor about what to expect during menopause and any new health concerns to watch out for. The more you know about this transition, the better you can handle symptoms and make smart choices about your health.
- **Embrace your authentic self:** Accept and appreciate yourself as you go through menopause. Feeling good about yourself comes from both your mindset and how you present yourself. Don't hesitate to do things that boost your confidence, whether it's trying new skincare routines or updating your wardrobe.
- **Let go of embarrassment:** There's no need to feel ashamed of menopause. Welcome this new phase of life as a celebration of being female, and don't let outdated ideas about aging stop you from living your life to the fullest.
- **Be flexible about your self-image:** As your body changes during menopause, be open to adjusting how you see yourself. Aging happens gradually, and it's okay if you don't look like the perfect images we see in the media. Focus on feeling healthy and confident in your own body.

Appreciate What You Have in Life

Instead of focusing on what you might be losing, think about the wisdom, experience, and freedom that come with age. Menopause can be a time for personal growth, self-discovery, and new opportunities.

Stay Confident

Keep your confidence up by taking care of your skin, staying active, eating well, and managing stress. Small changes in your daily routine can help you feel your best during this time.

In this chapter, we explored strategies for supporting longevity and aging gracefully during the menopausal transition.

As we move into the next chapter, our focus will shift to rebalancing weight management strategies during menopause. This is a critical consideration as hormonal shifts during this transition can significantly impact your metabolism and body composition.

6

REGULATING YOUR WEIGHT

As Samantha hit her late 40s, she began experiencing some unwelcome changes. The weight seemed to be creeping on despite her best efforts to control her diet and exercise regularly. She had always been able to maintain her weight relatively easily, but suddenly nothing was working for her. This frustrated her.

Samantha soon realized that the hormonal shifts of menopause were playing a role in what was happening to her. She was tired all the time, her cravings were all over the place, and that stubborn belly fat just wouldn't budge. Plus, her metabolism felt completely out of control.

Determined to regain her body and self-confidence, Samantha knew she needed to try something new. She started by focusing on gut health, incorporating more probiotic-rich foods and a targeted supplement into her routine. This made a huge difference. Not only did her digestion improve, but her energy levels also went up and she felt less bloated.

Samantha, with the help of a personal trainer, adjusted her exercise plan, placing more emphasis on strength training to counteract the muscle loss that her trainer warned could occur during menopause. Lifting weights became a game-changer for her. She felt stronger and more toned, and it really helped rev up her metabolism.

With these strategies in place, Samantha was able to shed the extra weight and maintain a healthy, comfortable size. Menopause definitely presented some new challenges, but by tuning in to her body's changing needs, she was able to find a sustainable approach that worked for her.

In this chapter, we'll dive into the sixth part of the 7 **RESTORE Steps to Gut Health**, which is all about **R**egulating your weight.

REBALANCING YOUR WEIGHT DURING MENOPAUSE

As we move into menopause, many of us find ourselves outsmarted by the frustrating challenge of weight gain. While it's true that our hormonal changes play a role in this process, all is not lost yet! The weight gained is not inevitable or permanent. We can take some proactive steps to regulate weight during this stage of our lives.

One general misconception is that solely being in menopause causes weight gain. While hormonal changes do influence weight, they're not the sole reason for weight gain. Lifestyle factors like diet and physical activity also play a great part in how much weight is gained and where those pounds choose to sit on our bodies. When we make healthy choices in these areas, we can effectively manage and reduce the weight gained during perimenopause and menopause.

You will need to handle weight management during menopause with a well-informed and holistic approach. Working with a healthcare professional can help you create a personalized plan that includes a balanced diet, regular exercise, and potentially weight loss medications if needed. HRT is just one potential approach to reaching a healthy weight in midlife, but lifestyle modifications are crucial strategies for long-term weight management.

HOW MENOPAUSE AFFECTS WEIGHT MANAGEMENT

Menopause is a natural change in a woman's life that brings big hormonal shifts, often affecting weight. Gaining weight during menopause is common, and understanding why can be helpful.

It's important to know why weight gain happens during menopause. As women get older, their estrogen levels drop, changing their metabolism. Estrogen helps control body weight by affecting how fat is stored. Lower estrogen levels can lead to the body holding on to more fat, especially around the belly. Also, the body burns fewer calories at rest as we age, which also contributes to weight gain.

Weight gain can start during perimenopause, the phase before menopause. This phase usually begins in a woman's 40s, but it can start earlier. Hormonal changes during this time can cause symptoms like irregular periods, hot flashes, and weight gain. Once menopause is reached, weight gain might become more noticeable if steps to prevent it aren't taken early. Less physical activity, diet changes, and stress can all contribute to this. As people age, they tend to lose muscle mass, which also slows down the metabolism.

Weight gain during menopause can have serious health risks. Gaining weight, especially around the belly, increases the chances of developing type 2 diabetes. This occurs when the body struggles to control blood sugar, which is worsened by extra weight.

Being overweight strains your heart, raising the risk of high blood pressure, high cholesterol levels, and other heart problems. High blood pressure can lead to various health issues, so managing weight effectively during menopause is important.

THE RELATIONSHIP BETWEEN GUT HEALTH AND WEIGHT DURING MENOPAUSE

Our gut is home to many tiny organisms called the gut microbiome. They play a big part in how our bodies digest food, control inflammation, and tell us when we're full or hungry. Some of these bacteria are good at pulling out calories from food, making it possible for us to gain weight, especially when our metabolism slows down in menopause.

When our bodies have too much inflammation, they tend to store more fat. Some gut bacteria make substances that help control inflammation, keeping it in check. If we lose these helpful bacteria, inflammation can rise, leading to weight gain.

Our gut bacteria also influence the hormones that control hunger and fullness. If these bacteria get out of balance, the signals that indicate hunger or fullness can get mixed up, and we may eat too much or too little. This can affect our weight, especially during menopause.

Importance of Gut Health During Menopause

Studies show that menopause-related changes in hormones can alter the types of bacteria in our gut, potentially causing weight gain (Liu et al., 2022). To manage weight during menopause, it's crucial to support our gut health.

Weight Loss and Gut Health

Research suggests that people who lose weight often have a diverse and balanced gut microbiome. Supporting gut health can also help with intestinal health, reducing problems like "leaky gut," which are linked to weight gain and inflammation.

Taking Action for Gut Health

During menopause, it's essential to take steps to support gut health. Keeping a food diary can help you see how your eating habits affect your gut and weight. Seeking advice from a health-care provider or a nutritionist can also give you personalized guidance on improving your gut health and managing your weight effectively.

WEIGHT MANAGEMENT TIPS DURING MENOPAUSE

Managing weight during menopause can be challenging. Women going through menopause experience hormonal changes that affect their metabolism, appetite, and fat storage. These changes can make weight loss more difficult. A key hormone during this phase is estrogen; as its levels drop, it can lead to an increase in the fat surrounding your organs, called visceral fat, which can be harmful to your health. Menopause often results in muscle loss and a slower metabolism, making weight management more of a struggle. Despite these difficulties, maintaining a healthy weight can offer various benefits to a woman's life.

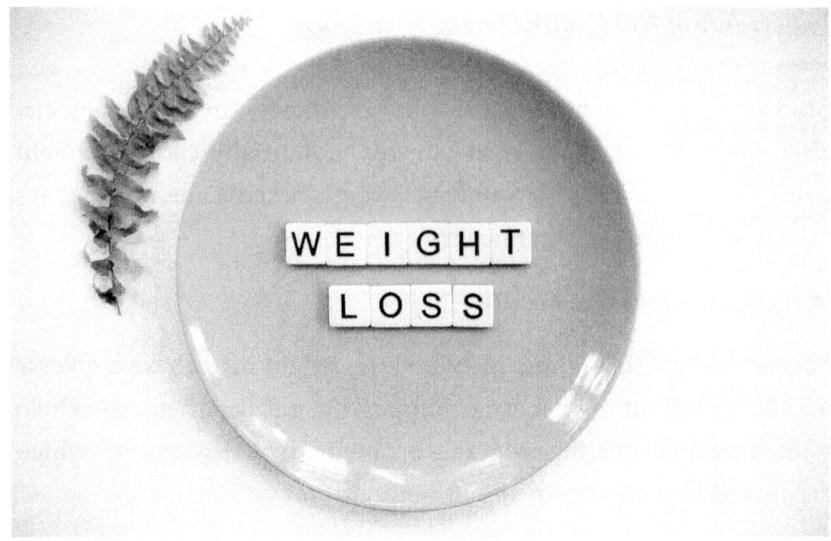

Limit Eating Sugary Foods

Sugary foods can lead to various health issues if consumed excessively. It's important to limit the intake of sugary foods to maintain good health and prevent problems like obesity, diabetes, and tooth decay.

Understanding Sugary Foods

Sugary foods are items that contain high amounts of added sugars, such as candy, soda, pastries, and desserts. These foods can be tempting due to their sweet taste, but it's essential to consume them in moderation.

Tips for Limiting Sugary Foods

- **Read labels:** When shopping for food, check the labels to identify products with high sugar content. Opt for items that are lower in added sugars.

- **Choose healthy alternatives:** Instead of sugary snacks, choose fruits, nuts, or yogurt as healthier alternatives. These options are still tasty but contain natural sugars and are better for your health.
- **Limit desserts:** Reserve desserts for special occasions and avoid consuming them daily. This can help reduce overall sugar intake and prevent cravings for sweets.
- **Drink water and unsweetened tea:** Sugary drinks like soda and sweetened tea are major sources of added sugars. Drink water as your primary beverage to stay hydrated without consuming extra sugar. If you like tea or herbal tea, try not to add any sugar.
- **Prepare meals at home:** Cooking meals at home allows you to control the amount of sugar added to your food. Choose recipes with less sugar and avoid adding extra sweeteners.
- **Practice portion control:** When indulging in sugary foods, practice portion control. Avoid eating large amounts in one sitting and savor small portions to satisfy cravings.

Impact of Limiting Sugary Foods

Limiting sugary foods can have positive effects on your overall health. By reducing your sugar intake, you may experience weight loss, improved energy levels, better dental health, and a decreased risk of developing chronic diseases like diabetes.

Maintaining a balanced diet with limited sugary foods is key to promoting a healthy lifestyle. By being mindful of your sugar consumption and making smart food choices, you can enhance your well-being and minimize the negative impacts of excessive sugar intake.

Boost Muscle Mass

Building up your muscle strength is a great way to help with weight management during menopause. Try incorporating weight-bearing exercises like lifting weights or doing squats. These exercises help maintain and grow your muscles, which in turn can speed up your metabolism to burn calories more efficiently.

Weight-Bearing Exercises

Incorporating weight-bearing exercises into your routine can contribute to building muscle mass. These exercises involve activities that make your muscles work against gravity, such as lifting weights and performing squats. By consistently engaging in these exercises, you can enhance your muscle strength, which is crucial for overall health and well-being during menopause.

Benefits of Muscle Growth

Building muscle mass offers various benefits besides weight management. It helps in increasing overall strength, improving posture, and enhancing balance and coordination. As muscles are metabolically active tissues, having more muscle mass can boost your resting metabolic rate, assisting in better calorie expenditure throughout the day.

Incorporating Strength Training

To effectively boost muscle mass, it is recommended to incorporate regular strength training sessions into your fitness routine. Strength training exercises target specific muscle groups and promote muscle growth over time. By gradually increasing the resistance or amount of weight used during training, you can continuously challenge your muscles and stimulate growth.

Progression and Variation

In your muscle-building journey, progression and variation are key factors to consider. Gradually increasing the intensity of your workouts and incorporating a variety of exercises that target different muscle groups can prevent plateaus and maximize muscle growth. Additionally, alternating between different types of strength training, such as bodyweight exercises and resistance training, can offer a well-rounded approach to building muscle mass.

Focus on Form and Technique

When engaging in weight-bearing exercises to build muscle mass, it's crucial to pay attention to proper form and technique. Ensuring that you perform each exercise correctly maximizes its effectiveness and reduces your risk of getting injured. Seek guidance from a fitness professional to learn the proper form for various exercises and make adjustments as needed to optimize your muscle building efforts.

Nutrition for Muscle Growth

In conjunction with strength training, proper nutrition plays a significant role in supporting muscle growth. Consuming an adequate amount of protein, which is essential for muscle repair and growth, is important. Including sources of lean protein in your diet, such as chicken, fish, tofu, and legumes, can help meet your body's protein needs for muscle development.

Rest and Recovery

Allowing your muscles time to rest and recover is equally important in the muscle-building process. Adequate rest periods between workout sessions enable your muscles to repair and grow stronger. Additionally, prioritizing quality sleep is essential as the body undergoes crucial repair processes while we sleep, including muscle recovery and growth.

Consistency and Patience

Building muscle mass is a gradual process that requires consistency and patience. By staying consistent with your strength training routine and making healthy lifestyle choices, you can effectively enhance your muscle mass over time. Celebrate small milestones along the way and remain dedicated to your fitness goals to experience the benefits of increased muscle strength during menopause.

Types of Exercises for Weight Loss During Menopause

Moving your body regularly is key to maintaining a healthy weight during menopause. Aim to engage in physical activities you enjoy, like brisk walking, swimming, or dancing. These exercises not only burn calories but also boost your mood and energy levels. Taking part in hobbies that make you happy can distract you from stress and emotional eating, contributing to better weight control and better mental well-being.

Aerobic Activities

When it comes to exercising to lose weight during menopause, aerobic exercises are effective. These activities get your heart rate up and can help burn calories. Examples of aerobic exercises include walking, jogging, swimming, or cycling. They are great for overall health and can contribute to weight loss by increasing your metabolism.

Strength Training

Strength training exercises are essential for women going through menopause. As we discussed in the previous section, building muscle can help boost your metabolism, making it easier to manage weight. Lifting weights or using resistance bands are good examples of strength training exercises. They not only aid in weight loss but also support bone health during this stage of life.

Yoga and Pilates

Engaging in activities like yoga and Pilates can be beneficial during menopause. These exercises focus on flexibility, balance, and strength. They may not directly lead to rapid weight loss, but they can help tone muscles, improve posture, and reduce stress— all of which are important for overall well-being during menopause.

High-Intensity Interval Training

High-intensity interval training (HIIT) workouts involve alternating between intense bursts of activity and short rest periods. This type of exercise can be effective for weight loss during menopause because it boosts metabolism and burns more calories in a shorter period. HIIT workouts can be tailored to personal fitness levels and are efficient for women with busy schedules.

Core Strengthening Exercises

Developing a strong core is important for overall health and can support weight loss efforts during menopause. Core exercises help improve stability and posture and can reduce the risk of injuries. Examples include planks, crunches, and leg raises. A strong core is not only aesthetically pleasing but also functional for daily activities.

Balance and Stability Training

As women age, balance and stability become increasingly important. Including exercises that focus on balance, such as standing on one leg or using a balance board, can help prevent falls and injuries. These exercises may not directly contribute to weight loss but are crucial for maintaining overall health and mobility during menopause.

Swimming and Water Aerobics

Swimming and water aerobics are low-impact exercises that are gentle on the joints, making them ideal for menopausal women. These activities can provide a full-body workout, improve cardiovascular health, and help in weight management. Exercising in water can also be a refreshing and enjoyable way to stay active during menopause.

Seek Professional Advice and Support

Don't be afraid to chat with your doctor about your weight goals during menopause. They can give you personalized advice based on your health needs and medical history. They might suggest specific strategies or treatments to help you manage your weight effectively. It's always good to have an expert in your corner when it comes to your health.

When considering hormone therapy to prevent weight gain, it's important to consult with a healthcare provider. Hormone therapy can help alleviate many menopausal symptoms, but it also comes with potential risks and side effects. The decision to pursue HRT should be based on a thorough discussion with your healthcare provider of the benefits and drawbacks specific to your health status and needs.

It's reassuring to know that menopause-related weight gain often stabilizes once the body adjusts to its new hormonal baseline. This doesn't mean weight loss will be effortless after menopause but rather that the rapid gains you might experience during the transition can level off.

Other Effective Diets for Menopausal Weight Loss

In Chapter 4, we discussed the menopause diet. Now, let's explore further examples of fostering a healthy diet.

Whichever you choose to do, fill your plate with lots of colorful fruits, veggies, lean proteins like chicken and fish, and whole grains. These foods are packed with good stuff your body needs without causing extra weight gain. Try to stay away from too many sweet treats as all that sugar won't help your waistline. Also, keep an eye on how much alcohol you drink; those calorie-laden drinks can sneakily pile on the pounds.

Low-Carb Diet

A low-carb diet is all about cutting down on carbs like bread, pasta, and sugar. You eat more protein and healthy fats to keep you feeling full and less likely to snack on unhealthy foods. This can help you lose weight by managing your blood sugar levels and making your body burn fat instead of storing it. It's like telling your body, "Hey, burn that fat for energy instead of storing it!"

Tips for a low-carb diet:

- Say no to sugary drinks and carb-loaded treats.
- Choose eggs, avocados, and nuts for quick and easy low-carb meals.
- Have a grilled chicken salad instead of a sandwich for a low-carb lunch.

Mediterranean Diet

We discussed the menopause diet in Chapter 4, which is based on the same principles as the Mediterranean diet. This is all about eating foods like fruits, veggies, whole grains, and lean proteins—think Greek salad with olives and feta cheese. These foods have nutrients that help keep your body healthy and reduce inflammation. It's like giving your body a dose of goodness to help manage your weight better.

Tips for the Mediterranean diet:

- Include colorful fruits and veggies in every meal.
- Season your food with herbs and spices instead of salt for extra flavor.
- Swap butter for olive oil when cooking for a healthier option.

Vegan or Vegetarian Diet

Going vegan or vegetarian means you skip meat and focus on plant-based foods like beans, lentils, and tofu. These foods are high in fiber and nutrients, which can keep you full and your weight in check. It's like loading up on the good stuff that doesn't weigh you down!

Tips for a vegan or vegetarian diet:

- Snack on hummus and veggies for a fiber-packed snack.
- Cook up a veggie stir-fry with tofu for a protein-rich dinner.
- Blend up a green smoothie with spinach and bananas for a nutritious breakfast.

The "Meno Belly" Diet

Menopause is a time when women experience many changes in their bodies. For some women, managing weight during this period can be challenging. One tailored approach to managing weight during menopause is the "meno belly" diet. This diet is designed specifically for menopausal women and focuses on foods that can help balance hormones, reduce inflammation, and improve gut health.

Benefits of the "Meno Belly" Diet

The "meno belly" diet offers several benefits for menopausal women. By incorporating foods that support hormone balance, such as leafy greens rich in vitamins and minerals, women can help regulate their body's hormone levels naturally. Lean proteins like chicken and fish provide essential nutrients while keeping you feeling full and satisfied. Additionally, fermented foods like yogurt or kefir can promote gut health, which is important for overall well-being during menopause.

Implementing the "Meno Belly" Diet

To start following the "meno belly" diet, begin by incorporating more leafy greens into your meals. Spinach, kale, and Swiss chard are excellent choices that can provide a range of vitamins and minerals. Include lean proteins like chicken, turkey, and tofu in your diet to support muscle health and reduce cravings. Fermented foods such as yogurt, kefir, or sauerkraut can introduce beneficial bacteria into your gut, improving digestion and overall health.

As you begin with the "meno belly" diet, it is essential to monitor your weight and overall health regularly. Keep track of any changes in your weight, energy levels, and overall well-being. If you experience any unexpected symptoms or concerns, consult with your healthcare provider promptly. Monitoring your progress can help you make adjustments to your diet and lifestyle as needed to support your weight management goals during menopause.

Stress Management Strategies for Controlling Weight

Finding ways to relax and reduce stress is super important for keeping your weight in check. When you feel stressed, your body produces more cortisol, a hormone that can lead to storing fat in your belly. To tackle this, try incorporating activities that help you unwind into your daily routine. You could try things like meditation to calm your mind, physical exercises to get your body moving, making sure you get enough sleep, doing hobbies you enjoy, hanging out with friends to boost your mood, and learning to relax with methods like deep breathing or tensing and releasing your muscles.

Mindfulness Meditation and Relaxation Techniques

Have you ever tried mindfulness meditation or deep breathing exercises? These methods can help you calm your mind and lower stress levels, which may help with managing your weight. When you focus on the present moment and take deep, slow breaths, you can feel more relaxed and less likely to grab an unhealthy snack.

The Connection Between Social Support and Sleep

As we mentioned in Chapter 5, having a strong social network can provide emotional support and encouragement on your weight-management journey—that's why we are restating its importance.

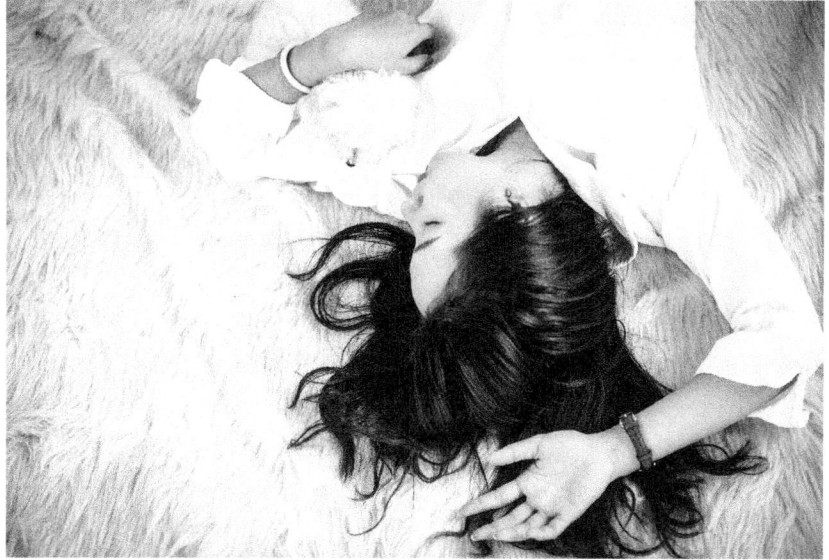

- **Social support:** Surrounding yourself with positive, supportive friends or family members can help you stay motivated and accountable. These relationships can also contribute to better overall well-being, including improved sleep habits.
- **Sleep:** Ensuring you get enough quality sleep is important for weight control. Lack of sleep can disrupt your hunger hormones, leading to increased food cravings and potential weight gain. Strive to get seven to nine hours of restful sleep each night to support your overall health and weight management goals.

A supportive social network can help reinforce good sleep habits and reduce stress, further aiding your weight management efforts.

Being well-informed and proactive about managing your weight during menopause helps you handle this stage of life better. Use the knowledge and tools provided here, and remember that small, steady steps can bring big improvements. Focus on a well-rounded approach involving diet, exercise, and lifestyle choices to pave the way for a healthier, more balanced life during and after menopause. Cheers to starting this journey with strength and positivity.

In the next chapter, we will embrace menopause and holistic gut healing as the last step in our RESTORE process.

7

EMBRACING MENOPAUSE AND HOLISTIC GUT HEALING

A ngela, a 55-year-old high school teacher, was known for her energy and enthusiasm in teaching. But when she started menopause, she faced hot flashes, mood swings, and trouble sleeping. Her doctor suggested hormone therapy, but Angela worried about the risks. Feeling desperate, she talked to her colleague, Maria, who had been through menopause.

Maria shared how she managed symptoms with a mix of treatments from a women's wellness center. Curious, Angela tried acupuncture, which helped with her hot flashes. She also did yoga and meditation, which improved her sleep and mood.

Over time, Angela felt much better. She even tried natural remedies that balanced her hormones. What she liked most was that the center focused on her overall well-being. She also joined a support group for women going through menopause.

After six months, Angela felt like a new person. She regained her passion for teaching and saw menopause as a time for self-discovery and greater health.

Menopause is a natural phase in a woman's life, but it's often misunderstood. It brings physical and emotional changes. Instead of fearing this time, we can see it as a chance for self-discovery and healing. Holistic health considers the whole person, not just symptoms, in order to take a more balanced approach to well-being. This chapter explores how combining modern medical treatments with traditional practices can help you through menopause.

Many women face challenges during menopause like hot flashes, night sweats, mood swings, and sleep problems. These issues can disrupt daily life, making women feel overwhelmed and alone. Some modern medical treatments like HRT come with risks like heart problems and breast cancer, causing women to seek safer alternatives. Holistic treatments, such as acupuncture, herbal remedies, yoga, and meditation, offer natural and effective ways to manage menopause symptoms.

In this chapter, we'll dive into the last part of the 7 **RESTORE Steps to Gut Health,** which is all about **E**mbracing menopause and holistic gut healing. We will explore the numerous benefits of holistic healing during menopause. You will learn about various natural treatments and lifestyle changes that can alleviate menopausal symptoms and enhance overall quality of life.

We will discuss how combining Western and traditional medical approaches can create a personalized, multifaceted treatment plan adapted to individual needs. When we explore these comprehensive strategies, you will gain insights into how to navigate menopause with greater ease, empowerment, and well-being.

THE APPROACH OF HOLISTIC HEALING

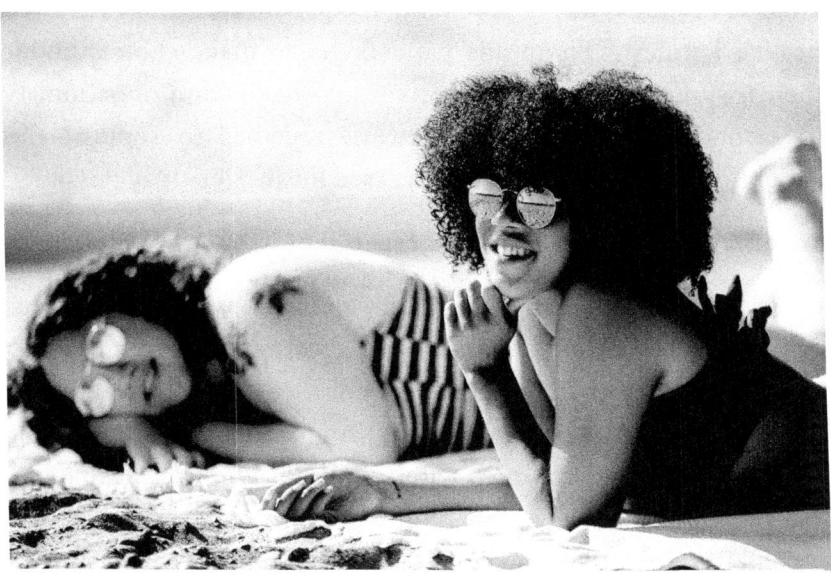

Holistic healing isn't just about treating the physical symptoms of menopause and gut health issues; it looks at how women feel emotionally and socially during this change. It combines old and new ways of healing to make sure women feel good all around. This kind of treatment takes a caring and strong approach, looking at all the different parts that make up a person.

Treating the "Whole Person"

When we talk about holistic healing, we mean treating the whole person—not just their medical problems. It's about making sure all aspects of a person's life are in balance. This may involve taking care of physical health, improving emotional and mental well-being, and helping someone succeed in their current stage of life. This can involve things like acupuncture, yoga, meditation, healthy eating, natural remedies, and counseling. All these practices aim to make sure a person feels their best inside and out.

Putting the Patient First

Holistic healing is all about making the patient a part of their own healing journey. This means patients get to make choices about their treatment. A team of experts from doctors and nutritionists to mental health professionals work together to support the patient. This ensures the patient is cared for in every way possible.

Benefits of Holistic Menopause Treatment

When we look at holistic treatments for menopause, we see why they might be better than hormonal treatments alone. Holistic treatments are tailored to fit each woman's unique experience with menopause. For example, herbal supplements like licorice, burdock, and others can help with symptoms without causing big changes in hormone levels. Eating foods with phytoestrogens like soy and flaxseed can help with hot flashes and mood swings.

Combine these supplements and foods with learning meditation and yoga to reduce stress levels. Holistic treatments are effective because our symptoms are often interconnected; for instance, increased stress will worsen gut health and hot flashes. Instead of treating a single symptom at a time, we should aim to improve the overall well-being of the person, which will help reduce their symptoms.

Feeling Stronger and More in Control

One big plus of holistic treatments is that they make women feel more powerful. When women take an active part in their treatment, they feel more in charge of their health. This includes both choosing treatments and making lifestyle changes like exercising regularly and managing stress. These changes can help with menopausal symptoms.

Getting to the Root of Things

Holistic treatments work well because they don't just cover up symptoms; they try to fix the cause of the problems. Things like acupuncture and yoga can improve physical symptoms like hot flashes and make a person feel more mentally clear and emotionally strong. By understanding that the body and mind are connected, holistic treatments can bring balance during menopause.

Interested in holistic healthcare options? You can find different professionals like naturopathic doctors, acupuncturists, and holistic nutritionists. Here's how to find the right provider:

- Start by researching certified practitioners in your area. Websites for organizations like the Cleveland Clinic offer directories of qualified holistic doctors.
- Look for providers who are members of reputable holistic medicine organizations as membership often indicates adherence to professional standards.
- Check online reviews and ask for recommendations from friends or family who may have had positive experiences with holistic treatments.
- Ensure that the practitioner is willing to communicate openly and respectfully about your health concerns and goals. Compatibility and trust between you and your provider are essential for effective care.
- Ask about their credentials, training, and experience in treating menopausal symptoms specifically.

BALANCING WESTERN AND TRADITIONAL REMEDIES FOR MANAGING MENOPAUSE

When dealing with menopause, using both Western and traditional medicine can give a well-rounded approach that respects personal choices while making the most of each medical style. Before we talk about how to integrate these treatments, let's see why this can be helpful.

On the one hand, conventional Western medicine offers several effective treatments, including hormone therapy, which has been shown to alleviate common menopausal symptoms such as night sweats, hot flashes, and bone loss (Ross, 2024). HRT can be tailored to individual needs, ensuring that women receive the support they require during this transition.

On the other hand, research indicates that hormone treatments come with serious risks, including a higher likelihood of blood clotting issues, breast cancer, and heart problems (Cho et al., 2023). However, traditional Chinese medicine (TCM) emphasizes holistic well-being and natural remedies, such as herbal supplements and acupuncture (Zhao et al., 2021).

Traditional and holistic approaches can complement Western treatments, offering a well-rounded strategy for managing menopause. For many, combining these methods results in optimal symptom relief and enhances overall well-being.

Combining Western and traditional treatments means integrating both to maximize their benefits. Here's how to approach it:

- Start by talking to a doctor who knows about Western medicine and a TCM practitioner. By working together, they can make sure to consider all aspects of your health.

- Use common medical tests to identify your specific hormone imbalances and other body issues. These tests can help decide what medications or treatments you might need.
- Use herbal supplements recommended by TCM, like black cohosh and dong quai, to naturally balance hormone levels. Always talk to your healthcare provider before taking these to avoid any problems with your prescribed medications.
- Try activities like yoga and meditation to help with stress and well-being. Both Western and traditional medicine approve of these therapies.

This two-pronged approach combines the benefits of Western medicine with the natural therapies and holistic philosophies of TCM. You can also try other types of alternative medicine like homeopathy and aromatherapy. Go to a licensed homeopath or aromatherapist for help.

Beyond integrating treatment methods, adopting a diet that supports overall health is another key element. We have explored various dietary recommendations for menopausal women throughout this book, and following those guidelines will further aid in holistically managing symptoms.

Natural Supplements for Managing Menopause and Gut Health

Let's explore some natural supplements known for their efficacy in managing menopause symptoms.

Black Cohosh

Black cohosh is an herb that many people find helpful for reducing hot flashes and night sweats, especially when taken along with St.

John's wort. Research has shown that it can also be beneficial for reducing feelings of depression often experienced during menopause (Shahmohammadi et al., 2019).

Red Clover

Rich in isoflavones, red clover acts like a plant-based estrogen called phytoestrogen. It can be useful for managing hot flashes without posing the same risks for breast cancer or heart issues that synthetic estrogens might.

Dong Quai

Often called the "female ginseng," dong quai is an herb commonly used in TCM for managing menopausal symptoms. It may work best when used in combination with other herbs and may be less effective when used alone (Johnson et al., 2019).

Maca

Originally from South America, maca root is known for its role in balancing hormone levels and boosting mood and energy. It can also help improve sexual function, which can be affected during menopause.

Soy

Adding soy products to your diet can provide natural estrogens that act similarly to human estrogen. This can help alleviate some of the hormonal symptoms associated with menopause.

Flaxseeds

Flaxseeds are a good source of lignans, which may help reduce the frequency of hot flashes and support heart health in general.

Ginseng

Ginseng is recognized for its energy-boosting properties and its ability to combat fatigue. It may also assist in managing mood swings and enhancing mental clarity during menopause.

Valerian

In cases where sleep problems are a major concern, valerian root can be a useful solution. It can create a sense of relaxation and improve the quality of sleep without causing the grogginess often associated with sleep medications.

Chasteberry

Effective in treating irregular menstrual cycles and premenstrual syndrome, chasteberry can also play a role in hormone balance during menopause.

Evening Primrose

Evening primrose oil contains gamma-linolenic acid (GLA), which may help decrease breast discomfort and the intensity of hot flashes.

Probiotics

These beneficial bacteria can help restore balance to the gut microbiome, which can be disrupted during menopause. They may improve digestion, alleviate bloating, and support overall gut health (Barrea et al., 2023).

Digestive Enzymes

Supplementing with digestive enzymes can aid in breaking down food, especially for those experiencing digestive difficulties during menopause.

Psyllium Husk Fiber Supplement

This is a type of fiber that takes in water in your digestive system, creating a thick gel. This can help you go to the bathroom regularly, ease constipation, and keep your gut healthy.

When picking a psyllium husk supplement, choose one that is pure and doesn't have extra fillers or artificial ingredients. Make sure you follow the recommended dose and drink a lot of water with it to prevent constipation.

Vitamin D

This vitamin is important for many body functions, including making hormones. Not getting enough vitamin D can lead to menopausal symptoms. The main way to get vitamin D is from sunlight, but some people might need supplements, especially in winter or if they don't get enough sun.

Omega-3 Fatty Acids

This is found in fatty fish, flaxseeds, and chia seeds. Omega-3 fatty acids can lower inflammation and help keep hormones balanced.

EMBRACING MENOPAUSE

Embracing menopause means accepting and celebrating this natural change in your life. It's more than just accepting it; it's about seeing menopause as a chance for growth, self-discovery, and empowerment, not something to fear. Menopause marks the end of being able to have babies, but it also starts a new part of our lives. This new chapter lets us focus on our well-being, dreams, and goals we might have put aside before. When we think of menopause positively, we can go through this time with more grace and confidence.

The Benefits of Menopause

Menopause has benefits too. You no longer have to deal with periods or worry about pregnancy. Many people also find that their sex drive increases during this time, leading to more intimacy in relationships. By focusing on these positives, you can change how you see menopause. One of the most immediate advantages is the cessation of menstrual periods. No more periods means no more cramps, PMS, or the inconvenience that comes with managing your monthly cycle. This physical relief alone can bring immense joy and freedom. Furthermore, the absence of periods eliminates the risk of pregnancy, which allows for a worry-free sexual relationship.

Beyond these tangible benefits, embracing menopause allows women to prioritize self-care, indulge in new hobbies, and redesign their daily habits to align better with their current needs and desires.

The Opportunity to Prioritize Self-Care

During menopause, taking care of yourself is very important. You need to listen to your body and understand what it needs. Self-care can be simple, like doing meditation or going for a walk. It's about making time for yourself every day, which can make you feel better overall. For example, set aside 10 minutes each morning to drink a cup of tea and relax. This quiet time can help start your day off positively and give you a moment to focus on yourself.

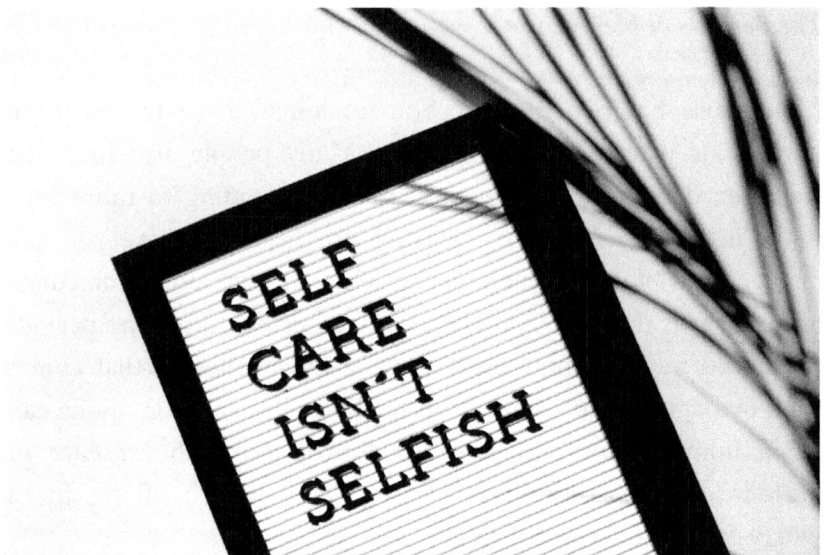

A Time to Take New Risks

Menopause is a time of change, and it gives you a chance to try new things. You might feel hesitant to take risks, but it can lead to personal growth. Trying something new, like learning a skill or traveling, can help you discover new interests and passions.

Steps:

1. Make a list of things you've always wanted to do but felt too scared to try.
2. Start with something small, like trying a new hobby or joining a class.
3. Reflect on how taking risks makes you feel and what you learn from the experience.

Redesigning Your Daily Habits

As you go through menopause, you may need to adjust your life-style to fit your changing body. This could mean eating healthier, getting more sleep, and staying active. These changes can help manage menopausal symptoms like hot flashes and mood swings.

An example of redesigning daily habits is incorporating more vegetables and fruits into your meals to support your body's needs during this time. Eating well can help you feel more energized and balanced.

Reflection and Personal Growth

Menopause is a good time to reflect on your life and think about your future. Journaling, talking to a therapist, or taking classes can help you grow personally and emotionally. It's important to make space for yourself to explore new ideas and feelings.

Steps:

1. Set aside time each week to reflect on your experiences and emotions.
2. Try different methods of self-reflection, like writing in a journal or having meaningful conversations with a close friend.
3. Consider what changes you want to make in your life and how you can work toward them.

No More Periods

One of the most immediate perks of menopause is the end of menstruation. The freedom from monthly bleeding isn't just a physical relief—it's a psychological one too. There's no need to constantly prepare for unexpected periods or deal with painful cramps and other premenstrual symptoms. The predictable absence of periods removes a persistent source of anxiety and inconvenience, allowing women to plan their lives without interruption. This newfound consistency can lead to a more relaxed and enjoyable lifestyle.

For example, think about how not having to buy tampons or pads every month can save you money and time. You can also enjoy the freedom of not being restricted by your menstrual cycle.

No More Pregnancy Risk

Another advantage is the elimination of pregnancy concerns. After menopause, there's no need to worry about contraception or the unanticipated consequences of intimacy. This can create a more spontaneous and carefree approach to sexual relationships. The peace of mind gained from this can significantly enhance your quality of life and sense of security. It's a unique freedom that deserves to be embraced and enjoyed.

Increased Sex Drive

Many women find that their sex drive increases after menopause. Freed from the fear of unintended pregnancies and possibly benefiting from a change in hormonal balance, many often rediscover or even heighten their sexual desire. This can lead to deeper emotional and physical connections with their partners, enhancing both the satisfaction and quality of intimate relationships. Experiencing a revitalized sex life can be one of the more delightful surprises of menopause.

Following these steps can help you make the most of menopause. Each woman's experience is unique, so talk openly with your healthcare providers to create a plan that suits you. Don't hesitate to ask questions, seek second opinions, and try different approaches for the best results.

Embracing menopause goes beyond just managing symptoms; it's about enjoying the freedom and new opportunities this phase brings. By taking care of yourself, being open to new experiences, changing your routines, making time for reflection, and focusing on the positives, you can navigate menopause with grace and excitement. Remember, this transition is a chance to discover new aspects of yourself and thrive in ways you never imagined. Feel free to explore some exciting herbal tea recipes included below before we continue to the Bonus Chapter.

HERBAL TEA RECIPES FOR MENOPAUSE RELIEF

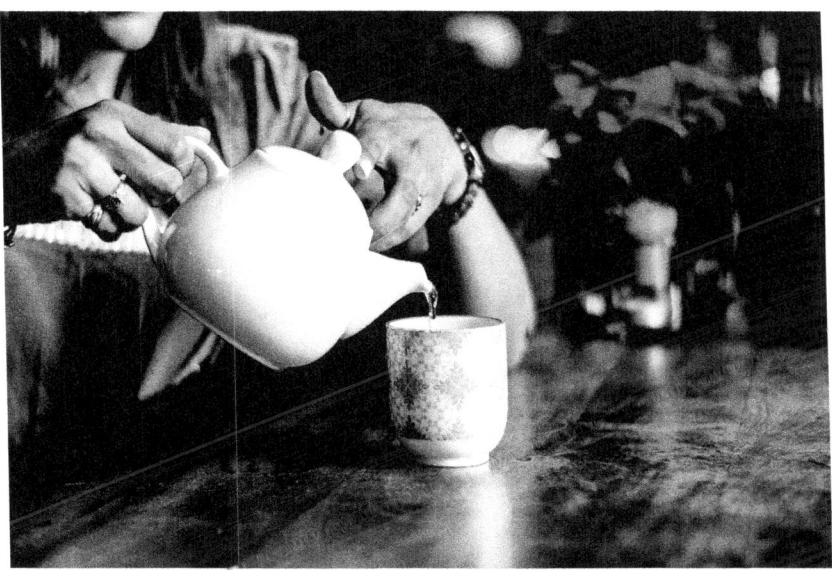

When managing menopausal symptoms, herbal teas can provide a soothing and natural approach. Drawing from empirical data and reflecting on the power of herbs, here are five herbal tea recipes that may alleviate common menopause symptoms such as hot flashes, insomnia, and anxiety.

Recipe 46: Black Cohosh Tea–Relief in a Cup

Ingredients & tools

- 1 tsp dried black cohosh root
- 2 cups water
- Honey or lemon (optional)
- Saucepan, strainer, and teacup

Instructions

- Boil 2 cups of water in a saucepan.
- Add 1 tsp of dried black cohosh root to the boiling water.
- Reduce the heat and let the mixture simmer for about 10–15 minutes.
- Strain the tea into a teacup.
- If desired, add honey or lemon to enhance the flavor.

Why it's beneficial

Black cohosh has been traditionally used to relieve hot flashes and night sweats, which are common during menopause. Some studies suggest it works by mimicking the effects of estrogen in the body, although more research is required to confirm its efficacy (Hill, 2020).

Recipe 47: Red Clover Tea–Natural Isoflavones

Ingredients & tools

- 2 tsp dried red clover blossoms
- 2 cups water
- Honey or mint (optional)

- Saucepan, strainer, and teacup

Instructions

- Boil 2 cups of water in a saucepan.
- Add 2 tsp of dried red clover blossoms.
- Let the mixture steep for about 5–10 minutes.
- Strain the tea into a teacup.
- Add honey or mint if you prefer a sweeter or fresher taste.

Why it's beneficial

Red clover is rich in isoflavones, compounds similar to estrogen, which may help alleviate symptoms related to declining estrogen levels such as hot flashes and night sweats (Dresden, 2021). While some studies have shown promising results, further research is still needed (Hill, 2020).

Recipe 48: Fennel Tea–Digestive Comfort and Calm

Ingredients & tools

- 1 tsp fennel seeds
- 2 cups water
- Honey or licorice root (optional)
- Saucepan, strainer, and teacup

Instructions

- Boil 2 cups of water in a saucepan.
- Crush 1 tsp of fennel seeds lightly with a mortar and pestle.
- Add the crushed seeds to the boiling water.

- Simmer on low heat for about 10 minutes.
- Strain into a teacup.
- Sweeten with honey or a small slice of licorice root if desired.

Why it's beneficial

Fennel boasts anti-inflammatory properties and can help with digestive issues often worsened by stress or hormonal changes. It also contains phytoestrogens, which might aid in balancing hormones during menopause (Dresden, 2021).

Recipe 49: Valerian Tea–Nature's Sleep Aid

Ingredients & tools

- 1 tsp dried valerian root
- 2 cups water
- Honey or chamomile (optional)
- Saucepan, strainer, and teacup

Instructions

- Boil 2 cups of water in a saucepan.
- Add 1 tsp of dried valerian root.
- Let it steep for about 5–10 minutes.
- Strain into a teacup.
- Add honey or a chamomile tea bag for extra relaxation.

Why it's beneficial

Valerian root is known for its calming effect, making it an excellent option for those struggling with insomnia or anxiety during menopause. It's been used historically to improve sleep quality and ease tension (Hill, 2020).

Recipe 50: Chasteberry Tea–Hormonal Balance Support

Ingredients & tools

- 1 tsp dried chasteberries
- 2 cups water
- Honey or lavender (optional)
- Saucepan, strainer, and teacup

Instructions

- Boil 2 cups of water in a saucepan.
- Add 1 tsp of dried chasteberries.
- Allow the berries to steep for about 10 minutes.
- Strain the tea into a teacup.
- Enhance the flavor with honey or a dash of lavender if desired.

Why it's beneficial

Chasteberry has been noted for its ability to influence hormone levels, potentially reducing symptoms like hot flashes and mood swings associated with menopause. However, it's important to note that some individuals may experience mild nausea or headaches (Dresden, 2021).

Through the thoughtful integration of these herbal teas, holistic healing becomes a comforting ally in navigating this life transition. While these natural remedies offer benefits, they should complement—not replace—conventional treatments.

———————

Let's move on to the bonus chapter where you will find valuable tips to help you continue on your wellness journey.

8

BONUS CHAPTER—CONTINUING
YOUR WELLNESS JOURNEY

Olga, a 53-year-old in marketing, was worried about menopause at first. Hot flashes made work tough, and mood swings strained her relationships. But after joining a support group, she saw menopause as a chance to grow. She added yoga to her daily routine, which helped with symptoms and her well-being. Now, Olga views menopause as a time for self-discovery and empowerment.

Another lady, Madelyn, a 49-year-old teacher, faced weight gain and fatigue during early menopause. Wanting to stay healthy, she talked to a nutritionist and started a Mediterranean-inspired diet. She also created a walking group with other teachers to mix exercise with social support. Madelyn's proactive steps didn't just help her handle menopausal signs but also led her to explore new interests like gardening and pottery.

Then there's Janet, a 56-year-old whose kids had left home and who felt adrift with the onset of menopause. Her doctor suggested she focus on her mental well-being, so she started journaling and practicing mindfulness. Janet also volunteered at an animal shelter, finding fulfillment in caring for others. The journey through menopause turned out to be a path to self-discovery and community involvement.

These three women's experiences show that menopause comes with challenges but also brings chances for personal growth, better health, and an enriched life. In this bonus chapter, we will recap the key points we've discussed and provide even more information to motivate you to continue with your wellness journey. We will explore a variety of strategies to support your health during menopause and beyond.

EMBRACING LIFELONG HEALTH

Stay healthy by taking care of your body, mind, and emotions. This means making choices like exercising regularly, eating well, resting enough, and practicing self-care. Being healthy is an ongoing journey, not just a one-time decision. This mindset can boost your quality of life, especially during menopause.

You have to focus on your physical and mental health as you get older. Physical health involves regular exercise, healthy eating, and seeing the doctor regularly, which can lower the chances of chronic diseases like heart problems, diabetes, and osteoporosis. For mental health, it's important to do activities that challenge your mind, reduce stress, and stay connected with others. Reading, puzzles, practicing mindfulness, and spending time with loved ones are all helpful. Adding these activities into your daily routine can help keep your brain sharp and your emotions stable as well as enhance your ability to cope with the challenges of aging.

Finding motivation to support lifelong health during menopause can be challenging but highly rewarding. To find motivation for supporting lifelong health during menopause, consider these strategies:

- **Set specific, realistic goals:** Break larger objectives down into smaller, more manageable steps. Instead of deciding to "eat healthier," start by aiming to add one extra serving of vegetables to your daily meals.
- **Build your support system:** Share your goals with friends or family members who can encourage you and hold you accountable. Consider joining a community group focused on healthy living or menopause support, which can provide camaraderie and support.
- **Celebrate small victories:** Reward yourself when you reach milestones, no matter how minor they may seem. Recognizing progress keeps you motivated.
- **Stay educated:** Reading up on menopause and health can empower you with knowledge and an understanding of your body's changes, making it easier to implement and stick to healthy practices.

Taking care of your health for life means consistently looking after your body, mind, and emotions. It involves making smart choices that keep you well, like exercising regularly, eating balanced meals, getting enough rest, and practicing self-care every day. This is especially important during menopause because it helps lessen the impact of hormonal changes and promotes graceful aging.

Focusing on lifelong health during menopause can help you better deal with issues like hot flashes, mood swings, and trouble sleeping. It also boosts your overall well-being, making you feel more confident and strong as you go through this stage. By paying attention to both your physical and mental health, you can lower your chances of encountering long-term health problems like heart disease, diabetes, and osteoporosis. You'll also keep your brain sharp and maintain emotional balance.

CONTINUING YOUR UNIQUE WELLNESS JOURNEY

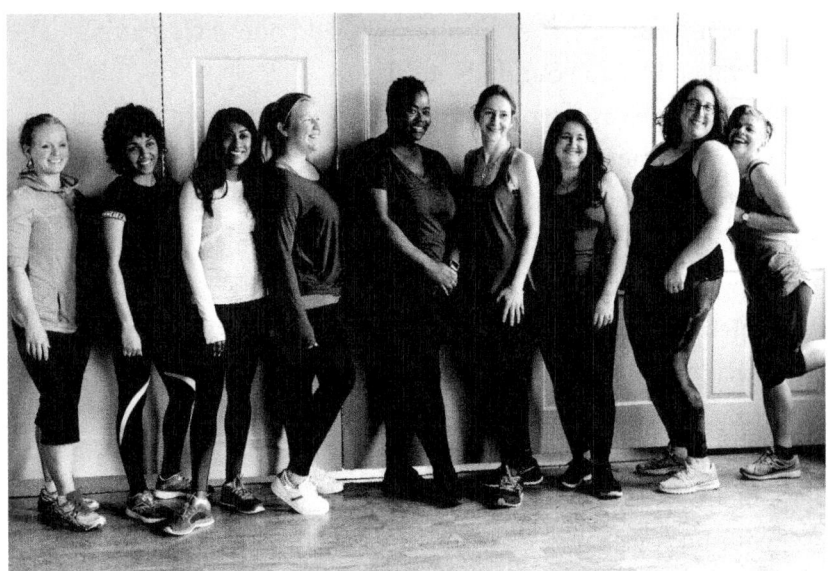

When you invest in your wellness during menopause, it helps you grow as a person. It allows you to learn more about yourself and take care of your mind, body, and soul. In this book, we've discussed ways you can do this. Let's review:

- **Get plenty of rest:** Establish a consistent sleep schedule and create a calming bedtime routine to combat sleep disturbances common during menopause.

- **Embrace mindfulness and meditation:** These practices can help you manage stress and foster inner peace. Start with short daily meditation sessions and gradually increase the duration as you become more comfortable.
- **Explore new hobbies:** Finding activities you're passionate about can bring joy and satisfaction, providing a creative outlet and a break from daily routines.
- **Incorporate self-care into your regular schedule:** Whether it's taking relaxing baths, practicing yoga, or reading, make time for activities you enjoy regularly.
- **Create motivational visuals:** Vision boards filled with inspiring images and words can keep you focused on your wellness objectives.

Self-reflection is important for supporting your wellness journey and personal growth. Writing in a journal regularly during menopause can help you learn more about yourself. Ask yourself questions like: What do I need right now? How have my needs changed? What is working well and what needs to change?

WORKING TOWARD WELLNESS GOALS

As you move forward in your wellness journey, let's reflect on the goals you set earlier. Remember those wellness goals from Chapter 2? Take a moment to revisit them. Look at how far you've come and consider what adjustments might be necessary as you continue to navigate your menopause journey.

Keep working on your wellness goals for your long-term health. Putting effort into these goals helps you stay ahead of any health issues and be ready for new challenges. Research shows that taking part in wellness activities can greatly improve your physical health and quality of life (*5 Tips for Setting Realistic Health Goals*, 2022).

Let's talk about how these goals can support your lifelong wellness. They serve as a framework that keeps you aligned with your values and needs, ensuring that you're always moving toward better health rather than stagnating or regressing. The act of setting and achieving these goals fosters resilience and adaptability, which are vital when your body is undergoing significant changes.

Examples of Goals for Each Health Category

Wellness encompasses various dimensions, each contributing to our overall sense of well-being. Let's explore the four main types of health and provide some examples of wellness goals in each category. Remember, committing to one small goal per category at a time can improve your life significantly.

Physical Health

Maintaining physical health is foundational to overall wellness. It's about keeping your body strong, flexible, and energized.

- **Example goal:** Aim to incorporate at least 30 minutes of physical activity into your daily routine. This could be anything from brisk walking to yoga sessions. Choose activities you enjoy and can sustain over the long term.

Mental and Emotional Health

Menopause can be a challenging time emotionally. Setting wellness goals that address mental and emotional health is key.

- **Example goal:** Practice mindfulness or meditation for 10 minutes each day. This can help reduce stress and anxiety to help foster a more positive mental state.

Social Health

Human connections play a vital role in wellness. Strong social ties can provide emotional support, especially during transitional phases like menopause.

- **Example goal:** Plan to meet up with friends or family at least once a week. Social interactions can boost your mood and provide a sense of belonging and support.

Spiritual Health

Spiritual health doesn't necessarily mean religious; it's about connecting with something bigger than yourself and finding meaning and purpose.

- **Example goal:** Allocate time each week to engage in activities that nourish your soul, such as journaling, nature walks, or attending spiritual services.

Use the below wellness goal planner to schedule your exercise session, meditation or mindfulness practice, social activities, hobbies or personal interests, and self-care routines in advance.

Wellness Goal Planner

Date: _____

Fill out this planner for each wellness category. Use a new planner for each month or quarter as needed.

Type of goal	Goal 1	Goal 2	Goal 3
Physical health			
Why it's important			
Action steps	1. _____ 2. _____ 3. _____	1. _____ 2. _____ 3. _____	1. _____ 2. _____ 3. _____
Deadline			
Status: Not started, In progress, Completed			
Type of goal	Goal 1	Goal 2	Goal 3
Mental and emotional health			
Why it's important			
Action steps	1. _____ 2. _____ 3. _____	1. _____ 2. _____ 3. _____	1. _____ 2. _____ 3. _____
Deadline			
Status: Not started, In progress, Completed			

Type of goal	Goal 1	Goal 2	Goal 3
Social health			
Why it's important			
Action steps	1. _____ 2. _____ 3. _____	1. _____ 2. _____ 3. _____	1. _____ 2. _____ 3. _____
Deadline			
Status:			
Not started, In progress, Completed			
Type of goal	Goal 1	Goal 2	Goal 3
Spiritual health			
Why it's important			
Action steps	1. _____ 2. _____ 3. _____	1. _____ 2. _____ 3. _____	1. _____ 2. _____ 3. _____
Deadline			
Status:			
Not started, In progress, Completed			

Creating motivational visuals can serve as constant reminders of your goals and progress. Vision boards filled with images and words that inspire you can keep you focused on your wellness objectives. These visuals not only motivate but also help to clarify what you want to achieve and remind you of the steps needed to get there.

Mindset Shift Exercise

Looking ahead, consider harnessing the power of self-reflection. Regularly evaluating your needs and strategies helps in adapting to new challenges. Writing down your thoughts and experiences can provide insights that guide your ongoing wellness journey. The knowledge gained from introspection will help tailor your approach, making your efforts more effective and personalized. Your path to wellness is ever-evolving, offering endless possibilities for enrichment and fulfillment.

Step	Action
Step 1: Identify a negative thought Think about a negative thought you've had about menopause.	Example: "Menopause means I'm getting old and losing my vitality." _____
Step 2: Challenge the thought Now, let's challenge this thought with evidence. Answer these questions:	1. Is this thought based on facts or assumptions? Or both? 2. What evidence contradicts this thought? 3. How might a friend challenge this thought if you shared it with them?

Step 3: Gather positive evidence

List three positive aspects or opportunities that menopause might bring.

1. _____

2. _____

3. _____

Step 4: Reframe the thought

Based on the evidence you've gathered, let's reframe your original thought into a more positive, growth-oriented perspective.

Complete the following sentence:

"Instead of [original negative thought], I can view menopause as an opportunity to..."

Example: "Instead of viewing menopause as losing vitality, I can view it as an opportunity to embrace a new phase of life with wisdom, freedom, and self-discovery."

_____

_____

_____

Step 5: Affirmation

Create a positive affirmation based on your reframed thought. Start with "I am..." or "I can..."

Example: "I am entering a vibrant new phase of life full of opportunities for growth and self-expression."

_____

_____

_____

Step 6: Reflection

How does this new perspective make you feel? What actions might it inspire?

Example: "This new perspective makes me feel hopeful and excited. It inspires me to explore new hobbies and prioritize self-care."

_____

_____

_____

This activity helps women challenge negative thoughts about menopause and see it as a way to grow personally instead of a setback.

Menopause is a new beginning. Use the advice from this bonus chapter to help you during this phase. Embrace your journey, celebrate your progress, and look forward to new adventures.

CONCLUSION

Menopause isn't a stopping point; it's a whole new chapter ready for you to explore and grow. Along the way, we've discovered how much potential menopause holds for change and self-discovery. It's about renewing yourself and uncovering new sides of who you are.

NURTURING YOUR GUT FOR OVERALL WELL-BEING

In our journey, we learned about the significant impact gut health has on managing menopausal symptoms. Think of your gut as a second brain, responsible for regulating hormones, digestion, immunity, and even mood. By giving your gut the attention it deserves—with a diet full of fiber, probiotics, and prebiotics—you're paving the way for reducing many common menopausal issues. Remember what we discussed: Simple adjustments to what you eat can lead to big improvements in how you feel every day.

Prioritizing Mental and Emotional Health

Taking care of your mental and emotional well-being is just as important during menopause as looking after your physical health. Mindfulness practices, like quiet reflection or jotting down your thoughts, can help you stay centered. Connecting with nature and spending time with loved ones can also boost your emotional strength through this transition. It's okay to feel anxious or blue; acknowledging those emotions and seeking support are vital steps toward navigating this phase with grace and resilience.

Embracing Your Unique Journey

Every woman's experience with menopause is different. The tips and suggestions shared here are only the beginning of your exploration. Trust your instincts, pay attention to your body's signals, and be open to trying new things to discover what fits you best.

Taking Action Toward Well-Being

Now is the time to put these learnings into practice. Pick one or two areas from what you've discovered that you want to work on and begin incorporating changes into your daily routine. Whether it's adjusting your diet, starting a new exercise regimen, or practicing mindfulness, consistency is key here. Celebrate even the smallest victories along the way as you progress toward a healthier you.

Seeking and Accepting Support

Throughout this book, we've seen the value of reaching out for help. Whether it's from professionals like doctors or nutritionists or sharing stories with other women going through the same journey, remember that you don't have to go through menopause on your own.

Support from others can offer comfort and invaluable insights that guide you as you walk this path. Similarly, supporting other women on their journey will empower you as well as help them find their way through menopause.

Stepping Boldly Into the Future

Menopause isn't solely about managing your symptoms; it's about flourishing and diving into this new phase with energy and confidence. You have the power to turn this transitional period into a period of growth, self-discovery, and improved health. Trust in your resilience, care for your body and mind, and step firmly into this exciting time of your life.

Welcoming Change With Optimism

As you close this book, remind yourself of the tools and knowledge you've acquired to support your well-being not just now but in the times to come. Have faith in your strength, nurture yourself, and move purposefully into this new phase.

The future holds so much promise; welcome this new experience with anticipation and curiosity. This is your opportunity to redefine what menopause means for you, changing it into a time of empowerment and positive change. Here's to your journey of rediscovery and renewed wellness!

TRANSFORM LIVES WITH YOUR REVIEW AND SHARE THE WEALTH OF WISDOM

Menopause is like a roller coaster for your body and mind. But guess what? We've got *The Ultimate Guide to Menopause Gut Health* to help you master this wild ride with a healthier gut and well-being. Now, it's time to guide others seeking the same triumphs.

Our mission is simple: to make menopause knowledge accessible to everyone. Everything we do revolves around that mission. And to achieve it, we need your voice—yes, yours!

Many people judge a book by its reviews, and your words can be the beacon of light for someone trying to navigate the choppy waters of menopause.

By sharing your honest thoughts about this book on Amazon, you're not just leaving a review but lighting the way for others searching for insights on menopause. You are extending a helping hand to someone out there who is in the same boat you once were. They are looking for answers, guidance, and a friend to help make menopause less of a mystery.

Your review could help...

...another woman embraces the journey of menopause.

...one more good friend trying to support her bestie through the changes.

... another woman to transit menopause into a period of growth and improved health.

....one more person to achieve holistic wellness and confidence.

It just takes less than 60 seconds to change another woman's life forever. To make a real difference, go to "Your Orders" in your Amazon account, choose the book, and click "Write a product review".

Thank you for being the bridge to knowledge. The world of Menopausal women thrives when we generously share our experiences, and your contribution is invaluable in keeping the flame alive.

Your partner in knowledge sharing,

Hera Bennett

PS - Did you know that sharing something valuable makes you more valuable to others? If you think this book will help another friend on their menopausal journey, pass it on. Sharing is caring!

ABOUT THE AUTHOR

Hera Bennett is a vibrant and insightful woman in her 50s and a mother of two daughters. She was a breastfeeding mother and certified consultant who helped many mothers breastfeed successfully. Now, she supports women in menopause as a continuation of her commitment to empower women.

Drawing upon her background working in women's health and wellness as well as extensive research, the author provides invaluable guidance to women facing the challenges of menopause. Hera is deeply committed to dismantling the stigma surrounding menopause and reshaping the narrative around this natural phase of life. Through her heartfelt books, she offers practical advice, evidence-based information, and emotional support that aim to ease the physical and emotional transitions during menopause.

Hera is a dynamic and compassionate author dedicated to empowering women who are navigating the transformative journey of menopause. Her warm and empathetic approach resonates with readers, making her a trusted voice in the realm of menopause literature. Through her books and advocacy, she encourages and inspires women to seek holistic well-being during menopause. Her mission is to empower women to embrace this phase of life with confidence and grace.

UPDATES FROM THE AUTHOR AND A CHANCE FOR A FREE BOOK

Let's celebrate menopause together! Join our mailing list and be the first to know about new upcoming books and receive updates and newsletters. You may even receive a FREE book!

To join our mailing list, email:

MenopauseWellnessBook@gmail.com

PS—Please add this address to your contact list to avoid emails going to the spam folder. Watch your inbox for updates and to see if you'll be receiving a FREE book!

ALSO BY THE AUTHOR

If you found *The Ultimate Guide to Menopause Gut Health* helpful in your menopause journey, consider reading the other published and upcoming books from Hera Bennett. Join our mailing list to receive updates whenever a new book is launched.

MENOPAUSE WELLNESS SERIES

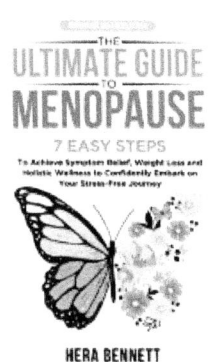

The Ultimate Guide to Menopause:

7 Easy Steps to Achieve Symptom Relief, Weight Loss, and Holistic Wellness to Confidently Embark on Your Stress-Free Journey

Audiobook available on Audible

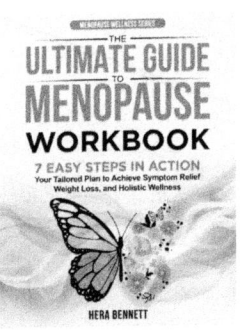

The Ultimate Guide to Menopause Workbook:

7 Easy Steps in Action: Your Tailored Plan to Achieve Symptom Relief, Weight Loss, and Holistic Wellness

Audiobook available on Audible

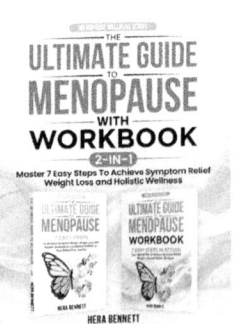

The Ultimate Guide to Menopause With Workbook 2-IN-1:

Master 7 Easy Steps To Achieve Symptom Relief, Weight Loss and Holistic Wellness

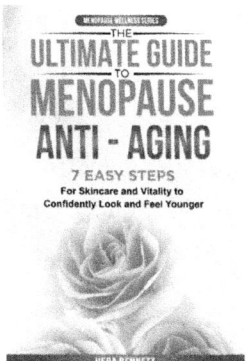

The Ultimate Guide to Menopause Anti-Aging:

7 Easy Steps for Skincare and Vitality to Confidently Look and Feel Younger

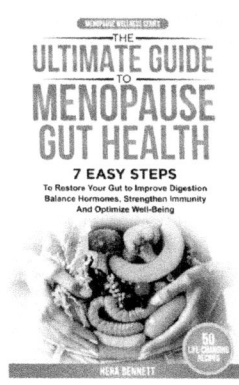

The Ultimate Guide to Menopause Gut Health:

7 Easy Steps to Restore Your Gut to Improve Digestion, Balance Hormones, Strengthen Immunity, and Optimize Well-Being

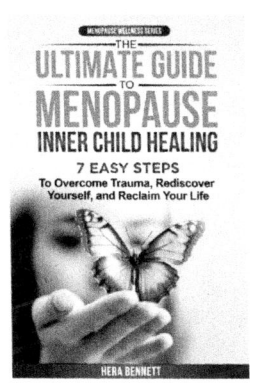

The Ultimate Guide to Menopause Inner Child Healing:

7 Easy Steps to Overcome Trauma, Rediscover Yourself, and Reclaim Your Life

PARENTING PERSPECTIVES SERIES

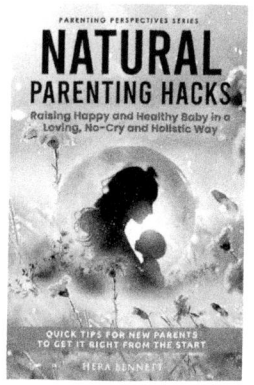

Natural Parenting Hacks:

Raising a Happy and Healthy Baby in a Loving, No-Cry, and Holistic Way. Quick Tips for New Parents to Get It Right From the Start

REFERENCES

Aspen Valley Hospital. (2023, June 29). *Mind your body: Embracing women's health, one healthy habit at a time.* https://www.aspenhospital.org/healthy-journey/mind-your-body-embracing-womens-health-one-healthy-habit-at-a-time/

Baker, J. M., Al-Nakkash, L., & Herbst-Kralovetz, M. M. (2017). Estrogen-gut microbiome axis: Physiological and clinical implications. *Maturitas, 103*, 45–53. https://doi.org/10.1016/j.maturitas.2017.06.025

Baothman, O. A., Zamzami, M. A., Taher, I., Abubaker, J., & Abu-Farha, M. (2016). The role of gut microbiota in the development of obesity and diabetes. *Lipids Health and Disease, 15*, 108. https://doi.org/10.1186/s12944-016-0278-4

Barrea, L., Verde, L., Auriemma, R. S., Vetrani, C., Cataldi, M., Frias-Toral, E., Pugliese, G., Camajani, E., Savastano, S., Colao, A., & Muscogiuri, G. (2023). Probiotics and prebiotics: Any role in menopause-related diseases? *Current Nutrition Reports, 12*(1), 83–97. https://doi.org/10.1007/s13668-023-00462-3

Barrow, D. (2023, January 4). *Yes, your gut health routine should change with menopause—Here's how.* Mind Body Green Health. https://www.mindbodygreen.com/articles/yes-your-gut-health-routine-should-change-with-menopauseheres-how

Bowel transit time. (n.d.). University of California San Francisco Health. https://www.ucsfhealth.org/medical-tests/bowel-transit-time

Bradley, C. (2024, March 12). *Reimagining your mid-life journey.* Mindful. https://www.mindful.org/reimagining-your-mid-life-journey/

Carr, A. C., & Maggini, S. (2017). Vitamin C and immune function. *Nutrients, 9*(11), 1211. https://doi.org/10.3390/nu9111211

CentreSpring MD. (n.d.). *How to test your gut function and evaluate your gut health.* https://centrespringmd.com/how-to-test-your-gut-function-and-evaluate-your-gut-health/

Charles Alexis, A. (2024, October 1). *6 filling parfaits that won't spike your blood sugar.* Healthline. https://www.healthline.com/nutrition/6-filling-parfaits-that-wont-spike-your-blood-sugar#6.-Berry-parfait

Chen, N. H. (2024, July 8). *Homemade miso soup (video).* Just One Cookbook. https://www.justonecookbook.com/homemade-miso-soup/

Cho, L., Kaunitz, A. M., Faubion, S. S., Hayes, S. N., Lau, E. S, Pristera, N., Scott, N., Shifren, J. L., Shufelt, C. L., Stuenkel, C. A., & Lindley, K. J. (2023). Rethinking menopausal hormone therapy: For whom, what, when, and how long?

American Heart Association. *Circulation* 147, Issue 7, 597–610. https://doi.org/10.1161/CIRCULATIONAHA.122.061559

Cirino, E. (2017, November 1). *Digestive health basics.* Healthline. https://www.healthline.com/health/digestive-health

Claudepierre, C. (2024, April 27). *Almond butter energy balls.* The Conscious Plant Kitchen. https://www.theconsciousplantkitchen.com/almond-butter-energy-balls/

Cole, J. (2023, March 16). *Quinoa vegetable salad.* Allrecipes. https://www.allrecipes.com/recipe/172050/quinoa-vegetable-salad/

Crichton-Stuart, C. (2023, January 12). *What are the benefits of eating healthy?* Medical News Today. https://www.medicalnewstoday.com/articles/322268#

Dalakas, K. (n.d.). *Strawberry overnight oats with honey and flaxseed.* Just a Pinch Recipes. https://www.justapinch.com/recipes/breakfast/other-breakfast/strawberry-overnight-oats-with-honey-and-flaxseed.html?r=19

Darnell, H. (2023, April 29). *Lemon tart: Healthy, beautiful & delicious.* Ancient Nutrition. https://ancientnutrition.com/blogs/all/lemon-tart

Dow, S. (2023, September 14). *Nutrition for menopause and perimenopause: Thriving through change.* Glacial Community YMCA. https://www.glcymca.org/thriving-through-change/

Dresden, D. (2021, December 23). *10 of the best teas to relieve menopause symptoms.* Medical News Today. https://www.medicalnewstoday.com/articles/menopause-tea

Edwards, A. (2023, August 14). *Almond buttercup green smoothie.* Belle of the Kitchen. https://belleofthekitchen.com/almond-buttercup-green-smoothie/

Escobar, S.-N. (2023, July 20). *The power of the Mediterranean diet for menopause.* Menopause Better. https://menopausebetter.com/mediterranean-diet-for-menopause/

Everlywell. (n.d.). 7 signs of a healthy gut + tips to improve digestive health. *Everlywell.* https://www.everlywell.com/blog/food-allergy/signs-of-healthy-gut/

Fable, S. (2016, January 15). *How to be consistent when working toward your wellness goals.* American Council on Exercise. https://www.acefitness.org/resources/everyone/blog/5802/how-to-be-consistent-when-working-toward-your-wellness-goals/

5 tips for setting realistic health goals. (2022, June 24). PeaceHealth. https://www.peacehealth.org/healthy-you/5-tips-setting-realistic-health-goals

Galloway, J. (2022, April 29). *3 under-the-radar signs you actually have great gut health.* Well+Good. https://www.wellandgood.com/signs-healthy-gut/

Goldman, R. (2023, May 30). *7 benefits of cucumber water: Stay hydrated and healthy.*

Healthline. https://www.healthline.com/health/food-nutrition/cucumber-water

Gut check: How the microbiome may mediate heart health. (2021, January 1). Harvard Health Publishing. https://www.health.harvard.edu/heart-health/gut-check-how-the-microbiome-may-mediate-heart-health

The Gut Health Doctor. (n.d.). *Is my gut healthy?* https://www.theguthealthdoctor.com/gut-health-quiz

Hartstra, A. V., Bouter, K. E. C., Bäckhed, F., & Nieuwdorp, M. (2015, January 1). Insights into the role of the microbiome in obesity and type 2 diabetes. *Diabetes care*, 38 (1): 159–165. https://doi.org/10.2337/dc14-0769

Hill, A. (2020, September 30). *10 herbs and supplements for menopause.* Healthline. https://www.mcmasteroptimalaging.org/full-article/wrr/10-herbs-supplements-menopause-769/website

How the bowel works. (n.d.). Bladder & Bowel Community. https://www.bladderandbowel.org/bowel/bowel-resources/how-the-bowel-works/

How to get more fibre into your diet. (n.d.). NHS. https://www.nhs.uk/live-well/eat-well/digestive-health/how-to-get-more-fibre-into-your-diet/

Jeyaraman, M., Ram, P. R., Jeyaraman, N., & Yadav, S. (2023). The gut-joint axis in osteoarthritis. *Cureus*, 15(11), e48951. https://doi.org/10.7759/cureus.48951

Johnson, A., Roberts, L., & Elkins, G. (2019). Complementary and alternative medicine for menopause. *Journal of Evidence-Based Integrative Medicine*, 24(1). https://doi.org/10.1177/2515690X19829380

Jolene. (2019, September 15). *Chia pudding with coconut milk recipe.* Yummy Inspirations. https://yummyinspirations.net/2019/09/chia-pudding-with-coconut-milk/

Kalra, B., Agarwal, S., & Magon, S. (2012). Holistic care of menopause: Understanding the framework. *Journal of Mid-Life Health*, 2(3), 66–69. https://doi.org/10.4103/0976-7800.104453

Kanakiya, A. (2024, January 24). Impact of stress on gut health during menopause. *Elda Health*. https://www.eldahealth.com/blog/impact-of-stress-on-gut-health-during-menopause

Koizumi, M., Ito, H., Kaneko, Y., & Motohashi, Y. (2008). Effect of having a sense of purpose in life on the risk of death from cardiovascular diseases. *Journal of Epidemiology*, 18(5), 191–196. https://doi.org/10.2188/jea.je2007388

Kresser, C. (2017, November 15). *The gut-hormone connection: How gut microbes influence estrogen levels.* Kresser Institute for Functional and Evolutionary Medicine. https://kresserinstitute.com/gut-hormone-connection-gut-microbes-influence-estrogen-levels/

Lamontagne, N. (2023, July 24). *Eight habits for longevity: Life-lengthening factors increase lifespan by 24 years.* Neuroscience News. https://neurosciencenews. com/longevity-lifestyle-changes-23685/

Larson, J. (2024, October 11). *Can menopause cause irritable bowel syndrome?* Healthline. https://www.healthline.com/health/menopause-irritable-bowel-syndrome

Leina. (2021, May 3). *Cinnamon ginger carrot muffins.* Tastes of Thyme. https://taste softhyme.com/2021/05/03/cinnamon-ginger-carrot-muffins/

Liu, Y., Zhou, Y., Mao, T., Huang, Y., Liang, J., Zhu, M., Yao, P., Zong, Y., Lang, J., & Zhang, Y. (2022). The relationship between menopausal syndrome and gut microbes. *BMC Women's Health, 22*(1), 437. https://doi.org/10.1186/s12905-022-02029-w

Lynch, S. V., & Pedersen, O. (2016). The human intestinal microbiome in health and disease. *New England Journal of Medicine, 375*(24), 2369–2379. https://doi.org/10. 1056/NEJMra1600266

Martineau, A. R., Jolliffe, D. A., Hooper, R. L., Greenberg, L., Aloia, J. F., Bergman, P., Dubnov-Raz, G., Esposito, S., Ganmaa, D., Ginde, A. A., Goodall, E. C., Grant, C. C., Griffiths, C. J., Janssens, W., Laaksi, I., Manaseki-Holland, S., Mauger, D., Murdoch, D. R., Neale, R., Rees, J. R., Simpson, S., Jr., Stelmach, I., Kumar, G. T., Urashima, M., & Camargo, C. A., Jr. (2017). Vitamin D supplementation to prevent acute respiratory tract infections: systematic review and meta-analysis of individual participant data. *The BMJ,* 356, i6583. https://doi.org/10.1136/ bmj.i6583

Mayo Clinic Staff. (2023, July 8). *The reality of menopause weight gain.* Mayo Clinic. https://www.mayoclinic.org/healthy-lifestyle/womens-health/in-depth/ menopause-weight-gain/art-20046058

Menopause (Holistic). (n.d.). PeaceHealth. https://www.peacehealth.org/medical-topics/id/hn-1041009

Menopause topics: Hot flashes. (n.d.). The Menopause Society. https://menopause. org/patient-education/menopause-topics/hot-flashes

Munn, C., Vaughan, L., Talaulikar, V., Davies, M. C., & Harper, J. C. (2022). Menopause knowledge and education in women under 40: Results from an online survey. *Women's Health, 18*(1), 1–16. https://doi.org/10.1177/ 17455057221139660

Munuhe, N. (2022, April 15). *The gut-brain connection diet: A simple guide (with a food list).* BetterMe. https://betterme.world/articles/gut-brain-connection-diet/

Must-try tips for setting (and accomplishing) your goals this year. (2024, January 4). *University of Colorado Boulder Health & Wellness Services.* https://www.colorado. edu/health/blog/goal-setting

Nie, X., Xie, R., & Tuo, B. (2018). Effects of estrogen on the gastrointestinal tract.

Digestive Diseases and Sciences, 63(3), 583–596. https://doi.org/10.1007/s10620-018-4939-1

Nile, S. H. (2015). The nutritional, biochemical and health effects of makgeolli —a traditional Korean fermented cereal beverage. *Journal of The Institute of Brewing,* 121: 457–463. https://doi.org/10.1002/jib.264

Ouwehand, A. C. (2017). A review of dose-responses of probiotics in human studies. *Beneficial Microbes, 8*(2), 143–151. https://doi.org/10.3920/BM2016.0140

Patino, E. (2023, June 12). *9 signs of an unhealthy gut and what you can do about it.* Everyday Health. https://www.everydayhealth.com/digestive-health/signs-of-an-unhealthy-gut.aspx

Paula. (n.d.). *Brain healthy stuffed avocado salad.* Call Me PMc. https://www.callmepmc.com/brain-healthy-stuffed-avocado-salad/

Petre, A. (2023, December 5). *Habits to form now for a longer life.* Healthline. https://www.healthline.com/nutrition/13-habits-linked-to-a-long-life

Phelps, T., Snyder, E., Rodriguez, E., Child, H., & Harvey, H. (2019, November 27). The influence of biological sex and sex hormones on bile acid synthesis and cholesterol homeostasis. *Biology of Sex Differences 10,* 52. https://doi.org/10.1186/s13293-019-0265-3

Pickford, L. (n.d.). *Sumac chicken & hummus wraps.* Taste.com.au. https://www.taste.com.au/recipes/sumac-chicken-hummus-wraps/541d4e84-75be-45e8-8c4d-be6f3287e3f0

Prasad, A. S. (2008). Zinc in human health: Effect of zinc on immune cells. *Molecular Medicine, 14,* 353–357. https://doi.org/10.2119/2008-00033.Prasad

Probiotic supplements dosage: How much is enough? (2019, March 12). *Specialty Enzymes & Probiotics.* https://specialtyenzymes.com/blog/probiotic-supplements-dosage/

Qi, X., Yun, C., Pang, Y., & Qiao, J. (2021). The impact of the gut microbiota on the reproductive and metabolic endocrine system. *Gut Microbes, 13*(1). https://doi.org/10.1080/19490976.2021.1894070

Raman, R. (2023, March 20). *12 foods that contain natural digestive enzymes.* Healthline. https://www.healthline.com/nutrition/natural-digestive-enzymes#TOC_TITLE_HDR_2

Robertson, R. (2023, April 3). *How does your gut microbiome impact your overall health?* Healthline. https://www.healthline.com/nutrition/gut-microbiome-and-health

Ross, V. K. (2024, April 30). *Navigating menopause: Signs, stages, and symptom relief.* Baystate Health. https://www.baystatehealth.org/articles/navigating-the-menopause-transition

Rossi, M. (2021). *Love your gut: An easy-to-digest guide to health and happiness from the inside out.* The Experiment.

Ruder, D. B. (2017). *The gut and the brain.* Harvard Medical School. https://hms.harvard.edu/news-events/publications-archive/brain/gut-brain

Santoro, N. F., Coons, H. L., El Khoudary, S. R., Epperson, C. N., Holt-Lunstad, J., Joffe, H., Lindsey, S. H., Marlatt, K. L., Montella, P., Richard-Davis, G., Rockette-Wagner, B., Salive, M. E., Stuenkel, C., Thurston, R. C., Woods, N., & Wyatt, H. (2022). Charting the path to health in midlife and beyond: the biology and practice of wellness. *Menopause, 29*(5), 504–513. https://doi.org/10.1097/GME.0000000000001995

Scanlan, T. (2021, June 21). *Eating for your heart: The Mediterranean diet.* Mayo Clinic Health System. https://www.mayoclinichealthsystem.org/hometown-health/speaking-of-health/eating-for-your-heart-the-mediterranean-diet

Schapowal, A., Klein, P., & Johnston, S. L. (2015). Echinacea reduces the risk of recurrent respiratory tract infections and complications: A meta-analysis of randomized controlled trials. *Advances in Therapy, 32,* 187–200. https://doi.org/10.1007/s12325-015-0194-4

Schimelpfening, N. (2023, July 24). *These 8 habits could help you live decades longer.* Healthline. https://www.healthline.com/health-news/these-8-habits-could-help-you-live-decades-longer

Shahmohammadi, A., Ramezanpour, N., Mahdavi Siuki, M., Dizavandi, F., Ghazanfarpour, M., Rahmani, Y., Tahajjodi, R., & Babakhanian, M. (2019). The efficacy of herbal medicines on anxiety and depression in peri- and post-menopausal women: A systematic review and meta-analysis. *Post Reproductive Health, 25*(3), 131–141. https://doi.org/10.1177/2053369119841166

Smiley, B. (2023, May 30). *How much fiber should I eat per day?* Healthline. https://www.healthline.com/health/food-nutrition/how-much-fiber-per-day

Summers, K. (n.d.). *Western vs Eastern medical treatments for menopause.* Clemson University. https://opentextbooks.clemson.edu/sciencetechnologyandsociety/chapter/chinese-medicine-in-womens-health/

Stewart, M. (2022, December 5). *How to stay positive during menopause.* National Council on Aging. https://ncoa.org/article/how-to-stay-positive-during-menopause

Strawberry kefir parfait (how to layer kefir). (n.d.). CulturedFoodLife.com. https://www.culturedfoodlife.com/recipe/strawberry-kefir-parfait-how-to-layer-kefir/

Tiralongo, E., Wee, S. S., & Lea, R. A. (2016). Elderberry supplementation reduces cold duration and symptoms in air-travellers: A randomized, double-blind placebo-controlled clinical trial. *Nutrients, 8*(4), 182. https://doi.org/10.3390/nu8040182

Tresca, A. J. (2023, May 18). *Your digestive system and how it works.* Verywell Health. https://www.verywellhealth.com/your-digestive-system-and-how-it-works-1941716

WebMD Editorial Contributors. (n.d.–a). *The digestive system: How it works.* WebMD. https://www.webmd.com/digestive-disorders/your-digestive-system

WebMD Editorial Contributors. (n.d.–b). *How your gut health affects your whole body.* WebMD. https://www.webmd.com/digestive-disorders/ss/slideshow-how-gut-health-affects-whole-body

Well.org. (2019, April 1). *Why gut health matters more than you think.* https://well.org/healthy-body/gut-health/

What you should know about your gut health. (2022, December 30). Cleveland Clinic. https://health.clevelandclinic.org/gut-health

Wilmanski, T., Diener, C., Rappaport, N., Patwardhan, S., Wiedrick, J., Lapidus, J., Earls, J. C., Zimmer, A., Glusman, G., Robinson, M., Yurkovich, J. T., Kado, D. M., Cauley, J. A., Zmuda, J., Lane, N. E., Magis, A. T., Lovejoy, J. C., Hood, L., Gibbons, S. M., Orwoll, E. S., & Price, N. D. (2021). Gut microbiome pattern reflects healthy ageing and predicts survival in humans. *Nature Metabolism 3,* 274–286. https://doi.org/10.1038/s42255-021-00348-0

Youkilis, R. (2016, August 5). *Upgraded avocado toast.* Your Healthiest You. https://yourhealthiestyou.com/upgraded-avocado-toast/

Zhao, F.-Y., Fu, Q.-Q., Kennedy, G. A., Conduit, R., Wu, W.-Z., Zhang, W.-J., & Zheng, Z. (2021). Comparative utility of acupuncture and Western medication in the management of perimenopausal insomnia: A systematic review and meta-analysis. *Evidence-Based Complementary and Alternative Medicine: eCAM.* https://doi.org/10.1155/2021/5566742

IMAGE REFERENCES

Adeoye, A. (2017, February 24). *Lady running in a park in London* [Image]. Unsplash. https://unsplash.com/photos/shallow-focus-photography-of-person-walking-on-road-between-grass-ljoCgjs63SM

Barbhuiya, T. (2021, November 19). *A person holding a plate with a sandwich on it* [Image]. Unsplash. https://unsplash.com/photos/a-person-holding-a-plate-with-a-sandwich-on-it-xs2rdwVoqks

Calvar Martinez, A. (n.d.). *Three people have fun on a beach photo* [Image]. Burst. https://www.shopify.com/stock-photos/photos/three-people-have-fun-on-a-beach

Farah. (n.d.). *Women sipping cocktails in a white room photo* [Image]. Burst. https://www.shopify.com/stock-photos/photos/women-sipping-cocktails-in-a-white-room?q=Women+sipping+cocktails+in+a+white+room+photo

Hansel, L. (2019, August 1). *Unknown person holding white ceramic kettle* [Image]. Unsplash. https://unsplash.com/photos/unknown-person-holding-white-ceramic-kettle-WgvTj1l6wps

Henry, M. (n.d.). *Hanging with friends on the beach photo* [Image]. Burst. https://www. shopify.com/stock-photos/photos/hanging-with-friends-on-the-beach?q= women+on+beach

Inouye, M. (2019). *Self care isn't selfish signage* [Image]. Pexels. https://www.pexels. com/photo/self-care-isn-t-selfish-signage-2821823/

LuckyHand2010. (2020, May 22). *Falafel, food, hummus image* [Image]. Pixabay. https://pixabay.com/photos/falafel-food-hummus-arab-5203362/

M4rtine. (2017, December 29). *Food, wrap, vegan image* [Image]. Pixabay. https:// pixabay.com/photos/food-wrap-vegan-snack-a-drink-3048691/

Olsson, E. (2018). *Flat-lay photography of vegetable salad on plate* [Image]. Pexels. https://www.pexels.com/photo/flat-lay-photography-of-vegetable-salad-on- plate-1640777/

Pflug, S. (n.d.). *Smiling strong women together* [Image]. Burst. https://www.shopify. com/stock-photos/photos/smiling-strong-woman-together?c=fitness

Winstead, T. (2021). *Pink and white heart shaped candy* [Image]. Pexels. https://www. pexels.com/photo/pink-and-white-heart-shaped-candy-7722921/

Pixabay. (2016). *Woman lying on beige faux-fur mat* [Image]. Pexels. https://www. pexels.com/photo/woman-lying-on-beige-faux-fur-mat-206396/

Pixabay. (2017). *Men's white dress shirt* [Image]. Pexels. https://www.pexels.com/ photo/men-s-white-dress-shirt-356040/

ponce_photography. (2016, May 15). *Muffin, cupcakes, homemade image* [Image]. Pixabay. https://pixabay.com/photos/muffin-cupcakes-homemade-pastry- 1390368/

Tankilevitch, P. (2020). *Stir fry vegetables and tofu on a ceramic plate* [Image]. Pexels. https://www.pexels.com/photo/stir-fry-vegetables-and-tofu-on-a-ceramic- plate-5848482/

Total Shape. (2019). *Scrabble pieces on a plate* [Image]. Pexels. https://www.pexels. com/photo/scrabble-pieces-on-a-plate-2377045/

Vaitkevich, N. (2020). *Lavender flowers on a jar of delicious dessert* [Image]. Pexels. https://www.pexels.com/photo/lavender-flowers-on-a-jar-of-delicious- dessert-5803161/

Verduzco, M. (2024, May 15). *A close up of food on a grill with cucumbers* [Image]. Unsplash. https://unsplash.com/photos/a-close-up-of-food-on-a-grill-with- cucumbers-_wDfBXHIjtY

Zimmerman, P. (2020). *Close-up photo of woman touching her abdomen* [Image]. Pexels. https://www.pexels.com/photo/close-up-photo-of-woman-touching-her- abdomen-3958569/

Printed in Dunstable, United Kingdom

64666664R00122